NURSING IN THE SEVENTIES

ANNE ROE
MARY SHERWOOD

NURSING
IN THE
SEVENTIES

Selected readings that present both the old
and new trends to help create better nursing care
for patients

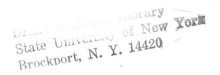
JOHN WILEY & SONS, INC.
New York London Sydney Toronto

Library of Congress Cataloging in Publication Data:
Roe, Anne K comp.
    Nursing in the seventies.

    1. Nurses and nursing — Addresses, essays, lectures. I. Sherwood, Mary, joint comp.
II. Title. [DNLM: 1. Nursing — Collected works. WY 100 R698n 1973]

RT63.R64   610.73'08   73-2874
ISBN 0-471-72962-0

Printed in the United States of America

10-9 8 7 6 5 4 3 2 1

PREFACE

Our purpose in selecting these particular articles are:

1. To make available information, opinions, and untested hypotheses that are not readily found in standard textbooks.

2. To broaden the reader's concept of how a nurse can be useful to a patient.

3. To show how patient care can be improved when a nurse thinks about it, researches it, and shares her findings and ideas with others.

We edited many of the articles for easier reading — not to change the authors' intent. For complete articles, see the source notes at the beginning of each selection and refer to the original publication. Some articles require the reader to take notes in order to keep track of the important points prior to the conclusion. Almost every article lends itself to individual or group discussion.

If you are an active nurse, you will find that many articles contain ideas that you will wish to incorporate into your present patient-care plans. Other articles may contain quick reference materials, such as the Fluids and Electrolytes chart on pages 242-243 and the list of Coping Behaviors on pages 157-158. Use the index to locate specific topics.

The articles are organized in five parts. Parts I to III discuss major topics: "Communicating"; "Knowing Your Ages"; and "Coping with Crises." These topics are especially useful in continuing your nursing education. Parts IV and V ("Some Basic Skills," and "Some Intensive Skills") discuss a variety of subjects — subjects that are of interest to beginning, intermediate, and advanced nursing students and practitioners.

We make short introductory comments at the beginning of each article, which explain why we feel that the article is important. The reader may perceive totally different ideas from ours, and this is highly commendable. Some readers are better listeners or viewers than they are readers and, for them, we have included some pointed questions at the end of each article. These questions should be read with a pencil in hand so that you can answer them while you are reading the article or after you have finished reading it. This will help you to understand the articles better.

More reflective questions also follow each article. These questions will help you to use the information in discussions, to transfer information contained in the readings to actual patient care, and to apply it while you are working with the nursing staff.

Many questions do not have easy answers but require you to think about the authors' statements. Then you must draw your own conclusions based on experience and knowledge. Do not become frustrated because you are not positive of only one "right" answer. Write out your ideas and answers so that you can use them in discussion groups.

Think about your own reaction to "unanswerable" or hard-to-answer questions. Why must you have an exact answer? Why don't you want the answer to be preceded by "If," "On the other hand," "Sometimes, but sometimes not," "It depends on," or in some way left open ended? When you look at life and nursing as it really is, you may find that there are not many questions that have exact and unchanging answers. We urge you to refer to these questions as you move from level to level during your nursing program and after graduation. Look back and see how your answers change as you change and mature.

We hope that this book will awaken both students and practitioners to the vitality, excitement, and possibilities present in nursing today. We view it as a supplement to the instructor and to the standard textbook — not as a replacement for either.

Anne Roe
Mary Sherwood

THE AUTHORS

ANNE ROE
R.N., B.S. Stanford University; M. Ed. Florida Atlantic University. Formerly instructor, Broward Community College and LPN program, Broward County, Fort Lauderdale, Fla.; office nurse, school nurse, and LVN instructor in California and Colorado.

MARY SHERWOOD
R.N. St. Luke's Hospital, Cleveland, Ohio; B.S.N., M. Ed. University of Florida. Formerly in-service director at Everglades Memorial Hospital, Pahokee, Fla.; instructor, Broward Community College, Fort Lauderdale; staff nurse and private-duty nurse in California, Ohio, New York, and Florida.

Mrs. Roe and Mrs. Sherwood are coauthors of the LEGS individualized learning system for nursing students, also published by Wiley.

ACKNOWLEDGMENTS

We are indebted to many warm human beings. We are especially grateful to the contributors, whose work makes possible stimulating learning experiences. We also thank unknown reviewers for their helpful criticism. We are particularly grateful to:

Kay Cheatwood	Our faithful "girl Friday, Saturday, Sunday. . ."
Malcolm Easterlin	Who encourages innovation
Suzy Lego	Who organized the source notes
Earl Shepherd	Who shared our vision

Finally we express our appreciation to the publishers and journals who have granted permission to use copyrighted materials in this fashion and thus make them doubly useful to students.

A.R.
M.S.

CONTENTS

xi

Part V   SOME INTENSIVE SKILLS

THE CONTRIBUTORS

Each contributor was asked to share information, feelings, or predictions about the future of nursing. Many of the contributors gave more information than is reflected in this list. To avoid repetition, these comments have been edited.

HELEN M. ARNOLD R.N., M.S. Assistant professor of psychiatric nursing at Adelphi University is the author of another article "I Thou" in the December, 1970 *AJN*.

HELEN W. ARNOLD R.N. Was a research assistant at Jefferson Davis Hospital, Houston, Texas when the article "Transition to Extra-Uterine Life" was written.

JOAN M. BAKER R.N., M.S. Post master's student in alcoholism nursing at the University of Washington. She enjoys working directly with patients in a psychotherapeutic counseling role and predicts that professional nurses will be working much more in the area of wellness and prevention.

BETTY LOU BARNARD R.N. Was head nurse in the intensive care nursery at Jefferson Davis Hospital, Houston, Texas when the article "Transition to Extra-Uterine Life" was written.

CAROL R. BAXTER R.N., M.S.N. Director of nursing, staff development at Children's Hospital in San Francisco. "I am attempting to innovate change in a community hospital; to update managerial performance; to effect improved delivery of care to our patients." She predicts nurses must become professional managers as well as professional practitioners of clinical nursing.

GWENDOLINE BELLAM R.N., M.A. Associate professor of nursing at Ohio State University predicts nurses will be more involved in health maintenance through community effort and through improved understanding of man as an individual and as a member of society.

MARGARET A. BERRY R.N., M.A. Was a doctoral student in cardiovascular physiology at the University of Colorado when the article "The Drops of Life: Fluids and Electrolytes" was written.

KARYL K. BLAIR R.N., M.S. is currently an active mother. While supervisor—director of public health nursing in Anoka, Minnesota, she implemented the concept of professional nursing contracts. She feels nurses need to be much more concerned about what the patient wants in health care and how we can cooperate with other helping persons to provide it and less concerned about preserving all our generally undefined uniqueness.

FLORENCE G. BLAKE R.N., M.A. Retired professor emeritus of pediatric nursing at the University of Wisconsin-Madison. She predicts nurses will become increasingly more competent with advanced education and clinical research and assume more and more leadership in development of ambulatory services for families.

RICHARD E. BURGESS B.A. Director of technical services at Pharmaseal, a division of American Hospital Supply Corporation. He has contributed educational efforts to help nursing adapt and use technological advances.

DORIS L. CARNEVALI R.N., M.N. Associate professor at the University of Washington school of nursing. She is coauthor of *Nursing Care Planning* and predicts increased skill, responsibility, and accountability for health care.

BETTY ANN COUNTRYMAN R.N., M.N. Assistant professor of maternal and child health nursing at Indiana University-Purdue University, Indianapolis Campus. She has contributed to the knowledge and techniques of breastfeeding and says, "I can't predict, only *hope* for increased emphasis on *preventive* health care and on-going investigation of the body's unique abilities to cope, naturally, with many of the problems confronting man's health."

MURDINA M. DESMOND M.D. Professor of pediatrics at Baylor College of Medicine.

RHEA FELKNOR A.B. Managing editor at *RN*. Although not a nurse, he has been a professional editor for health related publications for years.

MARY V. FENTON R.N., M.S. Assistant professor of nursing, Houston Baptist College specializing in respiratory nursing.

JEANNETTE R. FOLTA R.N., Ph.D. Assistant dean in the college of arts and sciences at the University of Vermont. She has contributed toward and is coauthor of nursing theory on death and dying. She predicts nursing will become more directed toward research and theory development.

GERTRUDE E. GIBBS R.N., B.A. Program director for Para Medical Occupations, Omaha Nebraska Technical Community College. She has written for the nursing literature in various fields.

NAOMI R. GILLIAM (BALLARD) R.N., M.A. Assistant professor at the University of Oregon school of nursing.

PHYLLIS GOLDIN R.N., B.S. Head nurse of the acute psychiatric ward at Brea Hospital, California. She predicts nursing will be unique among the professions; a helping profession based on social and scientific background.

JO ANNA A. GREEN R.N., B.A. In-service coordinator at St. Mary's Hospital, Saginaw, Michigan. She predicts a diminution of clamor about what nursing is, should be, or can be; "Nursing will focus on consumer of its services; will be more decisive in community health."

HELEN J. HAMES R.N., M.S. Associate professor of nursing at California

State University at Chico. She teaches an integrated course in the nursing care of the adult and child, viewing illness as it affects the individual and family. She predicts nurses will be actively involved in the innovative delivery of health care in a variety of settings with emphasis on prevention and the economically disadvantaged.

VERA HELLER (REYNOLDS) P.H.N., B.S. Liaison nurse for Contra Costa County Hospital, California. Her work makes continuity of health care possible through liaison activity between acute care institution and the community.

CYNTHIA H. HENDERSON (KELLY) R.N., M.S. Senior editor of the *American Journal of Nursing* predicts "fractionalization to extinction unless we use our only unique art, the intimate bodily care of the person as the vehicle to help him help himself."

JACQUELINE HOTT R.N., Ph.D. Associate professor at Adelphi University in the school of nursing has contributed "A Descartian philosophy—I think, therefore I am—plus a pediatric heart, soul and mind in a maternal body." She predicts that nurses are being freed to act more creatively—we should be doing more *with* consumers and *as* consumers of health care.

COLETTE B. KERLIN R.N., M.S.N. Associate professor of nursing at the University of Colorado has worked toward developing an integrated nursing curricula and in interesting students in maternity nursing. She feels nursing will continue to focus on care of people under stress of a health-illness nature with an increasing number of nurse practitioners in independent practice of health care, preventive and diagnostic.

JUNE S. LOWENBERG R.N., M.N. Part-time lecturer at University of California, San Francisco, plus working at home as mother, consultant, and writer. She is assisting nurses to deal with their own feelings as well as effectively helping patients cope with massive loss or death. She says "I believe that nursing must clarify, develop and communicate its unique contribution of 'care' in health and illness or we will continue to disperse energy without any effort. I would like to see nursing problems rather than the problems following from the traditional medical model."

JANET L. LUNCEFORD R.N., M.S.N. Instructor at the National Cancer Institute in Bethesda. She has developed an expertise in cancer nursing; has shared this with others in articles and meetings and with nursing students in work-study programs. She predicts the nurse will have more expertise and responsibility in the management of patient care.

GLEE GAMBLE LYON R.N., M.N. Now a fulltime wife and mother, she volunteers with a psychodrama group in her community. She is an experienced psychiatric nursing instructor.

ENID V. MCKINNEY R.N., M.S. LTC retired Army nurse and teacher. She predicts nursing will be nurse-directed, rather than doctor-directed, and that the roles of each are different but overlapping and cooperative. "I think nursing education is striving to help nurses become helping persons, with the ability to meet their own needs in more wholesome ways than by deriving their major satisfaction from their patients' dependence upon them."

WALTER MCQUADE. Member of the board of editors of *Fortune* magazine.

ELIZABETH JANE MEZZANOTTE R.N., M.S.N. Assistant professor and department chairman at University of Wisconsin-Milwaukee school of nursing. She considers her major contribution to nursing to be her daughter, who is a nurse, and her work involving patient teaching. She predicts more emphasis on health teaching and involvement of individuals in assuming responsibility for their health care.

FAY T. MOSS R.N., M.S. Was instructor in the school of nursing and research associate in the department of public health nursing at the University of North Carolina when the article "Confusion in the Management of Diabetes" was written.

JEANETTE NEHREN (CHAMBERLAIN) R.N., M.S. Chief of nursing and related therapeutic personnel section in the continuing education branch at the National Institute of Mental Health. She has done research and writing as a psychiatric-mental health educator and in continuing education. She predicts more specialization to further the nurse's own identity plus a forward movement generally based on a multidisciplinary approach to problem solving.

LOUELLA ILES NELSON R.N., M.A. Assistant professor in the department of nursing at College of St. Catherine, Gustavus Adolphus College, Minnesota. She teaches students about relating to people in an effective, helping way and predicts nursing must take a stand and emphasize its unique contribution to patients' welfare. "It's uniqueness lies in the nurse's individualized approach in helping the patient to deal better with current health crises and preparing him for the future."

MAJORIE E. NEWTON M.S. Assistant dean of academic affairs and associate professor of nutrition at the University of California school of nursing in San Francisco. She has contributed toward the nutrition component of nursing.

CONSTANCE NISSEN R.N., M.S. A certified nurse-midwife, associate professor at Northern Illinois University—nursing of maternal and child health.

HILDEGARD E. PEPLAU R.N., Ed.D. Professor, director of graduate program in psychiatric nursing at Rutgers University. She has contributed 25 years in graduate education in psychiatric nursing (1948-1973), which includes conducting clinical practice workshops for R.N.'s in the summer (every summer 1956-1969) in state hospitals across the nation. She predicts that nurses will secure autonomy in the practice of nursing and as coequal colleagues of other professionals in health care systems.

MIECZYSLAW PESZCZYNSKI M.D. Professor and chairman of the department of physical medicine at Emory University School of Medicine.

DONALD I. PETERSON M.D. Associate professor of pharmacology and assistant professor of neurology at Loma Linda University School of Medicine.

NORMA J. PETERS (THOMAS) R.N., M.N. Instructor part time at St. Anne's Hospital School of Nursing, Fall River, Massachusetts.

LYNN R. PURINTUN R.N., M.N. Assistant professor in the school of nursing at University California at Los Angeles. She predicts an expanded role for the nurse in delivering health care.

NANCY J. PUTNAM R.N. Was a research assistant at Jefferson Davis Hospital, Houston, Texas when the article "Transition to Extra-Uterine Life" was written.

KATE RANDALL REEVES R.N., B.S. Night supervisor, Childrens Hospital of Orange County, California. Her work includes supervising acute pediatric care, inservice, counseling, teaching, and liaison with medical students and house staff. She predicts "tracking or some form of internship to somehow separate the episodic and distributive forms of nursing, since one type of schooling just does not do it. Acute care nursing is becoming much too sophisticated for it not to be a specialty."

ETTA M. ROSENTHAL P.H.N., B.S. School nurse and winner of the Mary Roberts writing award of *AJN;* has published about one hundred articles. She predicts that nurses will be phased out to physicians assistants, and the like.

REVA RUBIN Professor and director of graduate programs in maternity nursing at the University of Pittsburgh.

ARNOLD J. RUDOLPH M.B.B. Ch. Was associate professor of pediatrics at Baylor University and director of the John A. Hartford Foundation, Inc. Transitional Care Nursery when the article "Transition to Extra-Uterine Life" was written.

BARBARA RUSSELL R.N., M.S.N., Assistant professor of nursing at California State College at Long Beach.

MARY C. SCAHILL R.N., M.S. Chief nursing consultant at the Eunice Kennedy Shriver Center. She teaches students "the importance of considering the child as a unique person whose rights to autonomy must be promoted."

NANCY V. SCHULTZ R.N., M.A. Instructor of parent-child nursing at Nassau Community College and is currently writing a book on problem solving in nursing. She predicts that nursing will begin to identify the health needs of people in the community as well as in acute care centers and intervene through anticipation of needs, prevention and health teaching.

BERNICE L. SHAW R.N. She is associate editor of "Group Practice" the Journal of the American Association of Medical Clinics.

CAROLE M. SHOCKEY. Captain, United States Air Force Nurse Corps.

SANDRA HATFIELD SNOW R.N., B.S. Teacher for the Carroll County Board of Education. Through defining the role of the CCU nurse she has participated in the evolving definition of today's nurse. She predicts that "the professional nurse will be primarily involved in patient teaching; this role will replace the skilled practitioner receiving today's emphasis."

KAREN C. SORENSEN R.N., M.N. Was instructor in nursing at the University of Washington at the time the article "A Patient's Concern With Death" was written.

ANTHONY R. STONE Ph. D. Associate professor of psychiatry at Johns Hopkins School of Medicine. With his background in psychiatric social work he has conducted seminars at all levels from students to assistant directors, introducing human relations concepts and enhancing communication skills within the discipline and across disciplines. He predicts nursing will be an indispensable art from the patient's point of view as it more actively reaches out to patients and their needs plus more status for patient care and programs improving this.

KATHE D.L. TEMPLE R.N., Ph.D. Associate professor of nursing at California State College, Bakersfield. She predicts that "nurses will realize that fatigue and boredom are the result of not being turned on by their job. Subsequently they will realize that to get turned on they must actively transact directly with patients. Then nurses will relearn or learn skills that put them in direct physical contact with patients."

OTTO F. THALER M.D. Professor of psychiatry at the Rochester School of Medicine.

PATRICIA R. UNDERWOOD R.N., M.A. Lecturer in the department of mental health and community nursing at the University of California at San Francisco; also a doctoral student in their nursing science program. She says, "The emphasis seems to be on accountability in terms of levels of education and possible entry into a career ladder. In practice, we are being asked to show differences between the results of A.A. education and B.S. education. For me this indicates a move toward basic nursing education during the first two years in higher education with an emphasis on generalization, with specialization coming at the B.S. and M.S. level. This also indicates to me that the technical nurse will develop more at the bedside, in-patient setting, while the professional nurse will develop more in the community health centers and other non-in-patient care facilities. I hope this means that some order will come to the chaos nursing education and service have been for so long."

GERTRUD B. UJHELY R.N., Ph.D. Professor, director of graduate program in mental health-psychiatric nursing at Adelphi University. She has developed a framework for nursing intervention based on a classification of experience.

JOEL VERNICK M.S.W. Clinical social worker, supervised intensive interviews with fatally ill children and explored the dynamics of crisis situations with nurses.

JULIA D. WATKINS R.N., M.P.H. Associate professor in the school of public health and the school of nursing, University of North Carolina. Her major contribution has been the "study of the home management of diabetic patients and preparing materials to be used in teaching; teaching public health nursing."

JESSIE F. YOUNG R.N., B.A. Teacher in intensive care nursing staff development, Toronto General Hospital. She founded the Canadian Association of Neurological and Neurosurgical Nurses Association.

NURSING IN THE SEVENTIES

The following poem reflects our philosophy — *Anne Roe, Mary Sherwood*

Those Young Nurses

Enid V. McKinney

My years show.
My grey hairs are many. Well earned.
I belong to "the establishment"
"The older generation"
And similar categorizations.
I don't mind.

I belong to the era
When a "good nurse"
Ran a "good ward."
Meaning the beds were neat
And all in a row;
The window shades at a precise level;
The bedside table devoid of all
But pitcher and neatly everted glass.
The patient clean, quiet
And mutely dependent.
"Routines" kept everything under control.
Busy feet and hands, and
Cool, closed lips indicated
The nurse was quite ideal.
That's the way I think.

It's downright embarrassing
To see a young, flip thing,
Cap a bit askew (if, indeed,
     she's wearing one at all!)
Hair tousled or wispy,
Or LONG! This slip of a girl
Comes to tell me that
The young mother, controlled epileptic
Is frightened about her new baby
And has been reassured that
She can call for help
Instead of walking to the nurses' station
In case of need. Indeed!
(Post-partum patients *ambulate*
And no nonsense about it.)

And what about that other?
Fresh-faced, glowing, soft of voice,
She disrupted the whole ward
By helping a mother nurse
Her babe the first time
Right at LUNCH HOUR!
Everyone'll be wanting, now,
To feed "on demand"
It's all right when they get *home*,
If they're determined on it.

What really plunges the scalpel
Deep in my professional pride
Is the way those patients bloom
And glow, and "settle down"
When these young idealists
Treat them. Amazing!
The "kooks," the troublemakers,
The "stupid ones"
Are smiling, grateful and more intelligent
Than I thought.

Oh, it's a painful sting
To witness the deft and gentle way
These youngsters are supplanting me!
My patients never lacked
A thing. I made sure of that!

Or did I really?
With shamed face
And not too good a grace
It's true—
I acknowledge and salute
The young, hip, brave and gentle
Ones who DO what nursing IS.

In time, perhaps, I'll learn
To nurse—and not to burn.

COMMUNICATING

The message in the preceding poem must be received and acted on. Instead of being possessive and defensive about their profession, the "good" nurses must open the doors to mutual understanding and growth.

The articles in Part I illustrate how the "old" (back rub and feeding) and "new" (touch and communicating) techniques work together to result in improved patient care. It is indeed difficult for the experienced nurse to learn new and different ideas and to change but it is also difficult for the new graduate, who is often made to feel inadequate because she is less experienced. Both types of nurses need and can learn from each other.

In this group of articles, you will read about a variety of patients — all with different problems, personalities, and in different settings but all requiring a nurse who can communicate. Some patients are in an intensive care unit, one is in a psychiatric setting, one is in her own home, and three are in general medical surgical units. As you will see, communicating with patients is one type of nursing treatment. As such, it needs to be recognized and described by those giving care; it needs to be included on the nursing-care plan; it needs to be reported on during the change-of-shift report; and it needs to be evaluated and described in the nursing notes along with the usual "Ate well, up for an hour." Sound impossible? These articles will show you some of the reasons for improving your communication skills as well as some practical skills. They will also give you a chance to try out some of your new ideas and skills on different patients.

As you read the first two selections you might want to take notes on WHY and HOW TO communicate.

The questions that precede and follow each article will help you to better visualize and understand the role of the nurse in each setting as a thinking, performing, and problem-solving health worker. No two situations are exactly alike to such a nurse, and this is the true challenge of nursing.

The public has become more conscious recently of body language that includes touching and the avoidance of touching others. In nursing, this act of touching other people plays a major role in the giving of physical and emotional care. Knowing the meaning behind touching gestures and the evolution of maternal touch gives the nurse a knowledge of what to observe and thus how to better help mothers and babies. Relief of pain and anxiety can often be obtained through touch when drugs have offered little solace.

Nursing is returning to the time when the giving of comfort to a person involved body contact and communication, and there was less reliance on medication. Research studies have shown how the patient who is actively involved in communicating with the nurse about his pain and pain-relief measures receives greater relief from his pain than the patient who is a passive recipient of medication. Reaching out to help such people involves our hands as well as our minds. Patients need a nurse who can break into their terrible isolation and use the ability to touch therapeutically.

TOUCHING

1.
Maternal Touch

Reva Rubin

TOUCHING EXPERIENCES

Before describing maternal touch, or more correctly, the development of maternal touch, let me evolve some approximation of a standard by which maternal touch can be measured. Some years ago, Margaret Mead produced a film showing how the women in some Polynesian culture went down to the waters, dressed in what nature had provided, to deliver themselves of their infants. In this film, a woman was seen making her way back to the beach within a few minutes of giving birth. She promptly proceeded to bathe her newborn infant. With Margaret Mead's voice extolling the truly maternal behavior, the new mother held her baby at arm's length from her own body, her arm firmly extended and rigid, her thumb locked under the infant's armpit and the rest of her hand rigidly propping his back at the shoulders. The infant's head wobbled, his legs hung downward, his free arm and legs flailed in midair, and his shrieks drowned out the film narrative extolling maternal behavior.

I doubt that we would accept this as a portrayal of either the ultimate or a standard of what we could term maternal behavior in touch. We might mumble something about cultural differences at this point to explain what seems inexplicable, but our own observations seem to give little support to cultural differences. On the contrary, we would classify this kind of touch as preliminary and predict that as this woman, regardless of culture, felt more comfortable about herself in this role-situation and in relation to this particular child, she would bring the child closer to her own body in a warmer, more encompassing manner.

This brings us to a statement of how a woman holds someone whom she loves. Such a statement is necessarily an idealized abstraction, but let us make

From "Maternal Touch" by Reva Rubin, published in the November 1963 issue of Nursing Outlook *Copyright © November 1963 by the American Journal of Nursing Company. Reproduced, with permission, from* Nursing Outlook.

one. A woman who loves must enfold the person she loves. Her upper arms and breast ache for contact. The action is impulsive and takes will power to inhibit. The impulse is to draw the person close in a tight embrace. You can check this against your own experience when you see a particularly adorable 2- or 3-year old child. What limits any overt expression in action of what you feel are considerations of one, how the child will respond and two, the appropriateness of such behavior on your part on the particular relationship you have with him. These considerations are present in a maternal-child relationship, also.

IMPULSIVE RESPONSE

If we can accept, tentatively, this statement of how a woman impulsively responds to a child that she finds lovable, then we must admit that we see no such response in a maternity ward or in a children's ward on the part of the mothers with whom we work. This is significant. We would have to agree with Levy that feelings of maternal love are not endowed, but are acquired over time and in experiences within the relationship of two people.

More than this, however, we may be able, through observation of the nature and kinds of maternal touch, to follow the course of the development of such a relationship. For those of us particularly interested in promoting and fostering this relationship, the nature and kind of maternal touch or contact permitted may serve as an index to the kinds of help our patients can use.

Specifically, in the beginning maternal relationship, as observed in the maternity wards, there is a definite progression and an orderly sequence in the nature and amount of contact a mother makes with her child. She moves from very small areas of contact to those more extensive. At first only her fingertips are involved, then her hands (including her palms) and then, much later, her whole arms as an extension of her body. The direction of contact areas is from the periphery of her body (note Margaret Mead's aborigine mother) inward, centripettally.

The rate of progression from one predominating form of touch or contact to another is dependent on how she feels about herself in this particular function of her role, on how she perceives her partner's (the infant's) reciprocal response to her, and on the character of the relationship at any given time. All three factors operate in determining the extent to which she dares permit herself to become progressively and more intimately involved.

The initial contacts made by the mother with her child are exploratory in nature. Fingertips are used predominantly, although the full length of the fingers are used also, but somewhat stiffly. This is not necessarily a graceless gesture. At this point, the mother will usually run one fingertip over the baby's hair, rather than her hand, to discover that his hair is silky. She will trace his profile and contours with her fingertip. If she turns his head toward food, she uses fingertips; if she has to support his head in bathing, she uses the index finger and thumb (no palm); if she has to turn him over, she seems to contact parts of him with her fingertips. She does use her arms and her hands to passively receive him, but her arms are not active participators in touch at this stage. Later, her arms will hold firmly, but just now she carries the baby as though he were a bouquet of flowers, in arms held so stiffly that she becomes fatigued.

EXPLORATORY CONTACTS

We use fingertips to explore, to obtain information. This is the tactile questioning we use in looking at a new piece of material, in making comparisons of quality, in determining when fruits are ripe. For purposes of important differentiation, fingertip touch is very valuable. And a new mother has some very important discernments to make in order to know with whom she is interacting as a mother.

In relationships between two people, fingertip contact is exploratory in nature. The person making the contact is not sure of how it will be received. This is true in courtship, before the handholding stage where mutuality has been established. In fingertip explorations, involvement is tenuous. In maternal touch, the fingertip stage precedes that of commitment.

Commitment seems to await some personally evocative response of the infant. Sometimes it is a burp, more often it is the particular way he cuddles, or, still more often, the way he expresses unbounded pleasure (three months later). This response must come from the baby, no one else, if this sense of partnership, of mutuality, in this kind of a relationship is to progress. The particular sign that satisfied the mother's requirements may vary. It should be pointed out that she is very vulnerable at this time to signs of rejection as well as responsiveness. But if the young mother has an essentially strong ego, she will search out, somewhat optimistically, positive signs of mutuality for a progressive relationship.

Yet to be fully verified is the impression that some mothers of children born with congenital handicaps are themselves handicapped in their maternal development by their babies' inability to respond normally. Specifically, and so far consistently, mothers of babies with hair lip and cleft palate seem to stay at the fingertip level of tactile interaction for a particularly long period. It remains to be seen whether response is sought primarily in the face and particularly in the mouth of the infant.

The next stage of maternal touch arrives gradually and is superimposed on the earlier stage. It is only by observing the same person over a time that one perceives a relative difference, but a significant one, in the manner of touch. The whole hand is used for maximal contact with the infant's body. The mother is more apt to support his entire buttocks in the cup of one hand. The hand on his back will be in full contact in every available surface of her palms and fingers. Both hands are relaxed and comfortable, representing how she feels about herself in her relationship with him. She transmits to him her security in herself through touch, and his responsiveness to her firm, comforting touch feeds back into her own well-being.

MATERNAL SELF-INVOLVEMENT

We see only the beginnings of this stage in the maternity wards. Somewhere between the third and fifth days postpartally, we see that she has advanced from fingertips to the whole-cupped hand to stroke her baby's head. She may start using the length of two or three fingers to turn his head. She begins to slip her whole hand under his back to turn him. But she still dresses him and bathes his rectum and genitalia by remote fingertips. Her arms and shoulders become progressively more relaxed and the distance between her body and that of the baby becomes shorter.

The changing body posture and the increasingly larger body surface involved in contact is indicative of an ongoing relationship in which the mother is becoming very much involved. It is at this time, no sooner, that she begins to ask realistic questions about his well-being and his care. At this time, she wants to assume a widening sphere of maternal functions, other than feeding. The content of her speech about him moves from the discovery and identification of him to self-involvement in his maintenance and care. Whereas before she would have informed us that "he spit up" and then dissociated herself from the event, she now responds directly to him by wiping him, changing his position, and comforting him (and herself). Her body language communicates symbolically that psychological work has progressed from the exploratory, information-seeking phase of an intimate relationship to that of involvement.

The multipara goes through these stages just as the primipara. Some multiparas do seem to move more readily from one phase to the next. Some of these, on follow-up, report ruefully that they moved too fast in assuming that one child was just like another.

Mothers who have had a very recent experience of appropriate and meaningful bodily touch from a ministering person, as during labor, delivery, or the postpartum period, use their own hands more effectively. This is true of both primips and multips. Conversely, if the mother's most recent experiences of contact in relation to her own body has been of a remote and impersonal nature, she seems to stay longer at this stage in her own activities with the baby.

I have not studied large numbers of maternity patients for as long as a year, but I have been struck by the very small percentage who, even at the end of a year, are sufficiently comfortable to hold their babies up close to their chests in pure enjoyment and pleasure in contact. I recognize that this is something of the moment and not sustained behavior. Those I have seen move on to this phase of contact with a baby under one year of age are those who enjoy contact, like mothers who really enjoy breast feeding and, of course, grandmothers and aunts.

Where I have observed mothers with hospitalized children under one year of age, I have been forcibly struck by the recapitulation of these stages in maternal contact, in the same ordering, particularly postoperatively. Maternal relationships are re-established first in fingertip identification, then in involvement of hands and then, very rarely, by the arms.

THE NURSE'S TOUCH

I would like to share some applications of touch for nursing, as an index of how a person feels about herself in an interpersonal relationship. Nursing students, like new mothers, are acquiring new roles and new identities. One of my faculty colleagues noted that the students' problem in timing contractions was due to their inability to make more than fingertip contact with the patient's abdomen. Shortly afterwards, I had the pleasure of supervising a group of basic students in the antepartal clinic, and one of my objectives was to help them discern approximate gestation, fetal position, and fetal heart rates. At the end of two weeks, they learned, through hearing, that the use of the entire hand surface provided more reliable information in palpation and that this was more comfortable to the patient.

But these are the so-called marginal learnings they made through touch: for them, raising a lady's skirt and slip was an appalling kind of behavior which was not in congruence with their concepts of how people should behave and not in accordance with their own self-concepts. This also applied to lowering the drape that exposes the upper fringe of a lady's pubic hair, as well as exposing her navel to public view and then participating in the viewing. Shame and confusion were the predominant feelings which they heroically tried to ignore. They felt that touching the flesh of another person intrudes on boundaries that are not to be violated. Nothing the patient, students, or I tried helped thaw the students' hands, which were stiff, awkward, cold, and useless. Probably nothing we tried was pertinent to what the students were experiencing. Skin, the students told me, is a strange thing; it is soft and rubbery; smooth and firm like marble, only warm. "It's warmer than you expect; sticky wet; feels doughy." "It's different."

How can you tell a young student that skin is all these things, but that it is something more? Is this not what she must learn for herself through touch, not words? When she has made her discoveries and made her inventory, she is ready to begin to function at a level we, and she, expect.

With unhampered growth, the beginning nurse and the beginning mother will develop their skills of information-gathering through touch into a source of discriminating for diagnosis and into a vehicle of personally meaningful communication. They will be able to read and recognize, through touch, the amount of body heat produced by a local or general body task; the kinds of perspiration produced by physical or psychological work. They will discern skin textures and recognize change, favorable or unfavorable. They will recognize another's appeal for contact, controls, or guidance, and be able to provide appropriate dosages of touch for each of these. And since touch is always individualized, the interpersonal communications effected through touch will tend to be significant in a way that verbal language cannot achieve.

Describe the stages of maternal touch that indicate that a new mother is accepting and mothering her new baby. What could you do to help her if, on the day of discharge, she still did not hold her baby close?

You might pass on the information to the office or clinic nurse so that the new mother will have continuing help and support as she learns how to touch and mother her infant. List some ways a nurse can help a mother during an office visit.

Do multipara's (mothers with more than one pregnancy) go through the same stages as primiparas (first pregnancy)?

How old is the infant before he can respond to a relationship with his mother?

In what way is a beginning mother compared with the beginning nursing student?

2.

The Back Rub

Kathleen D. Temple

Now that you are aware of the value and some meanings of touch, you can use the following article to learn some specific strokes useful when giving a back rub as well as applying the benefits you have learned about touch. Three purposes or benefits of giving a back rub are mentioned in this article. See if you can list them when you are through reading it.

The patient who spends most of the day and night in bed begins to use his back the way other people use their feet. But there is a great difference between the skin on the soles of our feet and the skin on our backs. The skin on the back is not prepared for the pressure of body weight and therefore requires the added nourishment of increased circulation.

Nurses employ the back rub as a part of the evening care which "settles the patient for sleep." Its soothing effect seems to relieve tension, thus promoting relaxation and sleep. It may also relieve headache due to tension in the neck and shoulders.

But nurses use the back rub for a third purpose, as well. A back rub is a physical measure but it can have a great emotional effect and can often be helpful in developing an interpersonal relationship with a patient. It provides that sense of touch which is in part responsible for the easy, quick rapport between patient and nurse that could take days if words alone were used.

One of the reasons some psychiatrists use a couch in treatment is to break eye contact between the patients and themselves. When a person is anxious it is difficult for him to express his anxiety or even to talk when he must by convention look at his counselor. All of us have seen the patient with rising anxiety who seems to need to break eye contact and will look down at his bedclothes or out the window; if this doesn't relieve his discomfort, the patient will usually change the subject. This problem of too much eye contact is resolved while the patient is receiving a back rub.

It is not only patients who become anxious in a nurse-patient relationship. Obviously, many situations arise in which nurses become anxious, too. Giving a back rub is physical work, and sometimes the nurse's anxiety can be dissipated by the physical labor. It is also a transition for the "doing" nurse who does not feel comfortable "just talking to patients." When a nurse cannot think of an appropriate response, the silence that occurs while she is thinking is not so traumatic when she is doing something. Even if she errs, cutting the patient off with a wrong response, the back rub will give her both the time and the opportunity to bring him back to the topic.

Similarly, the back rub can be used as a vehicle for conversation which helps in taking a nursing history. Even if the patient is tired of questions from the admission clerks and doctors, he will not mind giving information soon after he is admitted if the interview is pleasant and not like the question-and-answer session he's just been through. And, since a nursing history gathers information about things that are important to the patient's personal comfort, it will be easier for him than the other interviews—especially if a back rub is part of it.

Nurses sometimes say that there just is not time to give patients back rubs. Of course, seldom would there be time to give every patient a back rub. The nurse must choose, giving priority to those patients who most need time with her. Timing myself recently, I discovered that it took me 6 to 7 minutes to administer an oral analgesic and 10 to 13 minutes to administer a parenteral one. This time span included checking the last time the patient had the medication, signing out the narcotic, administering the medication, charting, and then checking to see the effect the medication had on the patient. The time we could save by giving back rubs would cut down on the time we spend giving analgesics and sedatives because, for many patients, the back rub will provide sufficient sedation and comfort.

There is no one technique for administering a back rub. In general, effleurage is a stroking motion, petrissage is a kneading motion, and tapotement is a tapping motion.

Whether a back rub will be sedative or stimulating depends on which of these motions predominates, the amount of pressure the hands exert, and the speed of the strokes. The back rub will be mainly stimulating if it consists of rapid firm strokes, using primarily petrissage and tapotement. There will be a sedative effect if more long slow stroking motions are used. If the back rub is intended to improve circulation, the strokes should follow the muscle in the direction of the return flow of circulation from the part. I have found the following back rub techniques useful for most patients:

1. *Effleurage.* This is a smooth long stroke moving the hands up the spine and then lightly down the sides to maintain contact with the skin.

2. *Pétrissage.* A large pinch of about three inches of skin and muscle is taken, moving up the sides of the vertebral column and then over the entire back.

3. *Tapotement.* The edge of the hand is used in a hacking motion over the surface of the back.

4. *Three-handed effleurage.* This is a smooth stroking motion I use which starts at the base of the neck and moves to the end of the shoulder. Before one hand leaves the shoulder, the other starts at the base of the neck, giving the patient a feeling of having three-hands moving. This is done on both sides of the neck, one side at a time. I usually complete the back rub with a light stroking movement over the entire back with the fingertips.

These methods of massage must be chosen carefully for each patient. Tapotement would not be used on an emaciated patient. Effleurage has to be adapted to a patient's needs. It can be done by exerting more pressure on the back of someone who is obese or muscular, or it can involve only the surface of the skin.

Each of these methods of massage should be used at least five times in order for the procedure to be called a back rub. Simply applying lotion on the patient's back without varying the methods of massage is an application of lotion, not a back rub.   In my experience, many patients have refused back rubs because they are both disappointed and uncomfortable when they get no more than cold, wet lotion on their backs.

The back rub offers satisfaction to the nurse as well as to the patient. The nurse, like the patient, has the satisfaction which touch adds to their rapport.

Moreover, the time spent in giving a back rub can be a relaxing moment during a busy shift. If she positions the patient well and assumes a relaxed position, using good body mechanics, the physical exertion is not great and, during this time, she is separated from the bustling activity on the ward. She is actually "busy with Mrs. Smith" so she is less likely to be interrupted than if she were "just talking with Mrs. Smith."

To sum up: Aside from the useful physical effects of the back rub, the act of giving it opens new channels of communication between patient and nurse as well as providing peaceful satisfaction for both.

Did you question how the nurse would remember or record the patient's answers given during a back rub? How much information can you retain when listening actively? One minute's conversation? Five minutes? If you were to use an observer to record the answers while you were giving the back rub, where would you instruct the observer to sit in relation to the patient if your patient were anxious? If the observer were anxious?

List four different strokes described in the article and indicate which strokes would not be used on an emaciated patient.

Note that the strokes are described in French terms. Try out each stroke as it is described so that your hands get the feel of what is being described.

Describe two different instances when a nurse might assign a nurse's aide to give a back rub to a patient and two other instances when the nurse would wish to carry out this procedure rather than delegate it to the assistant, and state why.

3.
Hospital Care of the Breast-Fed Newborn

Betty A. Countryman

You will find, in the next article, specific actions you can take to help a mother experience success in breast-feeding her infant while in the hospital.

A baby whose mother plans to breast-feed him needs, from the first moments after birth, different nursing care from that given to the baby whose mother plans to bottle-feed him.

THE FIRST FEEDING

It is common practice to offer glucose and water for the first feeding to the baby who will be given formula. This is said to be a precautionary measure in the event of esophageal anomaly. This feeding is given sometimes as late as 6 to 12 hours after birth. The breast-fed baby, however, does not need this precaution, since colostrum, a physiologic secretion, does not produce the irritating effects of a foreign substance.

A word about colostrum. It is considered by most authorities to be the logical first feeding of the infant. It is rich in vitamins A and E, high in protein, and contains immune factors. As the antibody content of colostrum is at its maximum during the first 12 postpartum hours, and as a baby's sucking reflex is strong immediately after birth, there should be little delay in putting the baby to the breast. Immediate feeding after birth will, in addition, help to establish the infant's early interest and coordination in suckling and provide him with valuable immunities. The first feeding should take place within the hour after delivery.

An additional benefit of colostrum is its laxative effect in the neonate. Early evacuation of meconium is thereby encouraged, making the baby hungry. The hungry baby is more likely to nurse vigorously at an early age, which stimulates the onset of lactation. In addition, the early evacuation of meconium tends to decrease the resorption of bilirubin from the cast-off red cells present therein.

LACTATION AND SCHEDULED NURSING

Nursing at four-hour intervals, has no valid rationale for the nursing mother. Such a schedule delays the onset of lactation. Additionally, it may pose problems of discomfort, even severe pain, for the mother if her milk comes in several hours before the baby is next permitted to nurse.

For the baby, a rigid schedule is equally inappropriate. The breast-fed baby's stomach generally empties sooner than does that of the formula-fed infant because of the finer curd and easier digestibility of mother's milk. The breast-fed baby therefore becomes hungry sooner than the bottle-fed baby and needs more frequent nursings.

Although frequent and early feeding usually brings in the milk within 36 to 72 hours, it is not uncommon for a mother whose infant nurses frequently on demand to have milk 24 to 36 hours after delivery. With the infant on a four-hour schedule, the first appearance of milk may be delayed until after the third day. Additionally, if the baby is not nursed during the night, the onset of lactation may be even later. The more the mother's breasts are stimulated, the sooner her milk comes in.

An additional disadvantage in scheduling nursing is that, because of ravenous hunger, the baby may voraciously suck and chew on the nipple, causing nipple pain and damage.

SUPPLEMENTARY FEEDINGS

The healthy breast-fed newborn when nursed on demand rarely needs supplementary fluid or nourishment. His mother's colostrum and milk generally provide adequate total intake. Water, plain or sweetened, dulls his appetite and diminishes or postpones his desire to suckle.

Since frequent and early feedings usually bring in the milk before the third day, the dehydration sometimes seen about this time is rarely encountered if the neonate is nursing adequately.

At any time, should it be necessary to give fluid other than from the breast, a spoon or eyedropper should be used.

Less strength is required for the baby to nurse from a nipple and he can become lazy at the breast if offered a bottle-and-nipple feeding.

DURATION OF FEEDINGS

A bottle feeding lasts as long as it takes the baby to empty the bottle or until he refuses it. Breast feeding differs in that a very intimate reciprocal relationship exists; the mother's comfort and condition require consideration along with the infant's needs. Special attention to the duration of each feeding must often be given for the first several days especially if a mother has not prepared her nipples prenatally. Because it is important that the integrity of the mother's nipples be maintained, it may be advisable to start with short nursings of about five to seven minutes, and increase their duration as the mother's tolerance permits. If the duration of nursing is limited initially, the frequency may be correspondingly increased to give the baby optimal total time at the breast.

Within a few days, when lactation is established, a baby's needs (tempered, of course, by the condition of the mother) will determine his particular frequency. The usual frequency is every two to four hours, with occasionally longer or shorter intervals between nursings.

The pattern of nursing also varies from baby to baby. Each infant early demonstrates his own pattern: some are vigorous, others dainty; some rapidly get to the business at hand, while others may dawdle or rest or play. An important point for the nurse is to recognize the pattern of the individual infant and permit him to fulfill his needs while assisting his mother to accept and feel comfortable with her baby's pattern.

NIGHT FEEDINGS

In many hospitals, bottle-fed infants are seldom taken to their mothers during the night. The breast-fed infant's night feedings, however, should not be omitted for the following reasons.

1. Frequent and regular suckling of the infant initiates an early, plentiful supply of his mother's milk.

2. The mother's milk may come in suddenly, and unless the baby nurses, the breasts can become overfull and rock-hard, and the baby may subsequently find it difficult or impossible to nurse.

3. The water which the infant may be given during the night if he is not put to breast tends to decrease his appetite and interest in sucking.

WEIGHT LOSS

The breast-fed baby who is nursed early and often, without regard for a schedule, rarely loses much weight. When his feedings meet his and his mother's needs rather than the arbitrary demands of hospital routine, the baby may reach or even exceed his birth weight by the third or fourth day.

Write an outline or a procedure for nursing care of breast-feeding babies and their mothers.

How long should a baby suck on each breast? Why?

How often should a baby be brought to the mother? qh? q4h? prn?

When should the first feeding occur?

What questions does the article leave unanswered for you? Write them down so you can refer to them later.

List the advantages of early breast feeding on a "demand" schedule.

List the benefits of colostrum to the infant.

THERAPEUTIC COMMUNICATION

4.

Talking with Patients

Hildegard E. Peplau

Describe, in writing, the purpose and value of your own conversations with patients.

Recall instances in which you felt uncomfortable, at a loss for words, or just plain anxious. Then recall situations with patients where you were quite at ease and conversation flowed easily. With these contrasting situations in mind, examine the specifics, such as:

- What was the subject of the conversation?
- Who was doing most of the talking and who most of the listening?

Now draw some conclusions.

- Do you hope the patient will chatter on about general topics?
- Do you habitually pause and ponder for maybe three to five seconds before you respond to what a patient is saying to you?

To pause and ponder requires practice and work but will be well worth the effort, when mastered, in your professional and personal life. We often jump in and make a reply without thinking of alternatives, especially when the topic or person is making us slightly anxious. The following article may motivate you to ponder your role in conversation.

Talking with patients is easy when the nurse treats the patient as a chum and engages in a give-and-take of social chit-chat. But when the nurse sees her part in verbal interchanges with patients as a major component in direct nursing service, then she must recognize the complexity of the process. Social chit-chat is replaced by the responsible use of words which help to further the personal development of the patient.

It is this complexity which distinguishes the verbal part of the professional nurse's work from the verbal approach a layman might use toward a sick person. The layman most often is actually a friend or a member of the patient's family, the nurse is a stranger to the patient.

There are marked distinctions between a layman talking to a friend and a nurse talking to a stranger who is a patient. The role of friend has its own requirements. Friends trust each other, exchange confidences, advise each other, lend one another money. Since it takes time for friendship to develop, two friends learn enough about each other so that behavior becomes predictable to a degree; one friend will begin to take certain actions of the other for granted. Acceptance of such assumptions is often the basis of meaning on which conversation between two friends is built.

The nurse and patient are not friends; they are strangers to each other. If the nurse does not see the patient as a stranger, about whom she knows nothing but can learn much, then she is distorting the facts of the situation. She can distort in different ways. She might look upon the patient as a friend, seeking in him familiar elements that she has previously experienced with friends in other non-clinical situations. Or she can look upon the patient in light of her own need or wish to have friends, thus relating to him primarily to fulfill her own wishes. Such wishes for friends ought to be realized in the social life of the nurse outside the hospital. Another distortion is for the nurse to see the patient as a disease category. In this situation she searches only for familiar clinical signs which help her to feel able, and she misses the unfamiliar, the unique newness of the *person* who is a stranger.

When the nurse treats the patient as a friend, she puts herself in the role of friend to him. The actions of the friendship role come to be expected of the nurse by the patient. Often the nurse burdens the patient with her biography, even sharing her secrets or seeking advice about her personal affairs. The focus on the needs of the patient is lost. Many nurses rationalize their actions along these lines, saying "it is good for the patient to take his mind off himself." If this be the case there are innumerable non-personal subjects of common interest which might be a more useful focus for social conversations with patients than the personal life of the nurse.

When the nurse sees the patient as a stranger, her first verbal task is to help him get oriented to her, to the hospital, and to the tasks at hand. Here, the layman in the nurse often gets in the way. To get oriented to a stranger outside the hospital, most people use social chit-chat at first. The questions go something like this: "Where do you live, Mrs. Jones?" "Have you lived there long?" "Do you know Mrs. Smith down the street?" "She went to Jersey High School, did you?" "I did too; did you take cooking with Miss Main?" and so on. The process is largely one of locating common if elementary interests and experiences as a base from which friendship might later develop.

This approach works well among laymen. The professional nurse, however, is offering a direct and specialized experience from which, hopefully, the patient will learn something of lasting personal value with regard to health. The professional nursing focus is the needs of the patient. The relationship, if it is to be governed by sustained objectivity in the interest of the patient's learning, will be time-limited by the duration of the illness—it is a temporary, often brief relationship. The approach to the stranger must therefore be different in the nursing situation.

THE PATIENT IN FOCUS

When the focus is on the needs of the patient, then the time of the nurse must be used purposefully in the patient's interest. This is not to say that the nurse does not have needs. Of course she does, for she is human too. But her needs are met outside the sickroom. Inside the sickroom, the focus is on the patient.

In getting oriented to the nurse, the patient needs to know her name, he needs to know that she is a registered nurse, what she may be called upon to do, the time limits which govern the duration and frequency of his contacts with her, and what she will do with information which she gets from him.

The patient may need validation of the self-evident. If he says "You have red hair" and the nurse has red hair, she can say "Yes, I do." But the patient does not need to know that all the women in the nurse's family for five generations back had red hair. If the patient notices a wedding ring on the nurse's finger and asks "Are you married," the nurse can reply "Yes, I am." But when she begins to describe the data and circumstances of the marriage this indicates pretty clearly that she is more interested in talking about herself than she is in the patient.

The nurse's biographical data is a burden to the patient who has no recourse but to translate the nursing situation into a social, chum-like one. Often the patient asks about the nurse's background primarily to test her capacity to focus on his needs and to find out whether she prefers instead to talk about herself. Since the patient must depend upon the nurse for many things, he will try to meet her needs so that he can feel safe with her. The nurse who can survive the patient's testing, and let him know clearly, simply, and directly that "this time is yours," will have offered the patient a unique experience with potential for learning.

Nurses should distinguish between a patient's demands and his needs. A demand is a request, a claim, or coercion to evoke some kind of response. In recognizing a need, on the other hand, the nurse draws her inference not only from such demands as the patient might make but also from her own observations and from other data.

A nurse does not meet the demands of a patient unless a valid need is represented in the demand. When a patient demands or asks persistently for biographical data from the nurse, she does not need to be pulled willy-nilly by these demands. She can say, quite simply, "Use this time to talk about you." Or she can ask gently, "What do you need this information for?" If the patient persists, the nurse might become more firm and ask, "Of what benefit to you would a review of my social life be?" or "I wonder what uses you would have for such personal information?"

Of course, if the nurse is desperate for the patient's approval and uncertain about her professional role and its boundaries, then she will simply yield to the patient and answer any and all questions about her personal life. In a general hospital no great trauma will thereby accrue to the patient; only another opportunity for a patient to learn something of value about himself will have been missed. In psychiatric work, however, the nurse will have proved to the patient his belief that people are not interested in him—only in themselves.

If the nurse wishes to focus on the needs of the patient, then she must know how to listen and how to respond in ways that will further the patient's learning. There is a technique for creative listening. It is not just a matter of letting a patient ramble on as though the nurse had her hearing aid turned off. It is more like listening to music—for the themes and variations, for the nuances of meaning that are conveyed indirectly through sound or hint.

Teaching a nurse to listen can only be done in clinical seminars, where interfering factors in the individual can be revealed and looked at and, hopefully, deleted. But there are some general guidelines.

Patients frequently make such comments as "I'm not hungry," "I'm not sleeping," "I'm not feeling well," or "I'm not comfortable." In situations such as these the verbal response of the nurse should be used to help the patient describe what went on instead of opening further discussion of what did *not* occur. Comments such as "What did go on" (instead of sleep), "What do you feel," or "Are you saying you are uncomfortable" help the patient to think directly about what did happen or is occuring.

In these situations, the nurse often automatically asks "Why not?" More often than not a "why" question has an intimidating effect. It has a ring of familiarity and is frequently reminiscent of earlier experiences when mother or teacher reiterated "Why don't you do this" or "Why can't you tell me" or some similarly coercing "why" question. Moreover, if the patient knew why he wasn't hungry or sleeping or comfortable, he would most probably deal with the situation. A "why" question asks for reasons which the patient is not likely to know immediately. He can discover them with help. But, in order to discover them, the patient requires some raw data—he must recall, for example what actually went on, instead of sleep. The reasons can be generalized from these data; then the "why" question can be answered.

PERCEPTIVE DESCRIPTION

In order to understand the reasons for the patient's behavior, both the nurse and the patient must have descriptions of the patient's experience. Such descriptions are not as easy to secure as many nurses assume. A great many people are singularly lacking in skill, especially in describing personal perceptions of experience.

Many nurses themselves do not describe what they observe but record instead stereotyped clichés which condense and classify rather than describe their observations. Valuable data from which fresh insight about illness could be drawn are lost this way. Verbatim descriptions given by psychosomatic and psychiatric patients would provide nursing with a far more useful base for determining nursing practice than the current tendency to translate doctors' findings into nursing knowledge.

Such words as "what," "where," "when," and "who" will assist the nurse to elicit useful description. A few highly serviceable clichés like "Tell me about that," "Then what," "Go on," and "You will remember" will be convenient when a direct question seems inappropriate. Except in rare instances, the nurse will find patients eager to talk about themselves; when a patient is reluctant or definitely not eager, the nurse can show respect for privacy of thought and silently await initial comments from him.

Words such as "how" or "why" are quite challenging ones. Nurses who really consider their meaning use them sparingly. The nurse who asks a patient "How do you feel" really asks, in effect, "In what manner or by what process do you have a feeling?" It would be simpler and more direct to ask "What are your feelings this morning?" The phrase "how come" is a cliché that communicates even less about what the nurse is seeking. In general, "how" and "why" questions require the patient to analyze the data of his experience and to respond with a generalization about it.

TROUBLE WITH PRONOUNS

"We," "they," and "us," are similarly troublesome pronouns.

Here is an example of a nurse reinforcing a patient's difficulty through the use of language:

A nurse said to a patient, "Let's go over what's been said and see if we have anything particular for us to discuss." The patient replied, "Oh, well, let's see what we'll see. Shall we watch for whether we are anxious between now and next week?" The merging of identity of nurse and patient—so that neither has the status of an independent person—is clear in this verbal interchange.

Magical or automatic knowing causes another communication problem. Magical knowing refers to knowing automatically—without asking, investigating, or finding out. Such phrases as "I know," "I see," "I understand" are included in this category when they precede rather than follow inquiry into a situation. Value terms such as "nice," "good," "bad" can also be used in such a way that consensus as to their meaning is assured rather than determined. For example, a patient said, "Well, last time my visitors were nice." The nurse responded, "Maybe today will go as well." This kind of verbal exchange shows the same limited communication inherent in such meaningless transactions as "Hello, how are you" to which the equally noncommunicative reply is "I'm fine, and you," and the final response is "I'm okay." Nothing has actually been said; these are merely words in juxtaposition.

The use of "they" as a pervasive global reference in which the identity of the referents is lost is typical of the patient diagnosed paranoiac. If you ask, "Who are they" the patient not only cannot tell you but may become quite anxious. If the nurse persists in asking, the "they" will become "other people," then a class of people as "my family" or "nurse" or "doctors," and finally names of particular people. Nurses should help more people become aware of the tendency toward loss of the referents by questioning "Who are they" whenever this pronoun is used.

SUMMARY

Talking with patients becomes productive when the nurse develops awareness of her own verbal patterns and then decides to take responsibility for her part in verbal interchanges with patients. When nursing is seen as an opportunity to further the patient's learning about himself, the focus in the nurse-patient relationship will be upon the patient—his needs, his difficulties, his lacks in interpersonal competence, his interest in living. What the nurse chooses to talk about during the relationship will be guided by her understanding of the scope and boundaries of nursing practice as a professional service.

Describe aloud or in writing three benefits to the patient that can occur from therapeutic communication with a nurse.

List three ways a nurse can distort her relationship with the patient.

State four "serviceable clichés" that Dr. Peplau suggests using to encourage patients to talk about themselves.

What alternatives does Dr. Peplau give for asking "Why?" after a patient's comment? Respond to the comments included in the article in alternate ways.

Dr. Peplau states that "Words such as how or why are quite challenging ones." Perhaps that is the reason for using the "how" and "why" between teachers and students and reserving the other, "softer" questioning pronouns for patients.

5.

Therapeutic Communication

Phyllis Goldin
Barbara Russell

Nine years elapsed between the writing of the preceding article and the next one. Much resistance to using "communication skills" instead of "just talking" with patients has been overcome and the general subject of hearing what patients are trying to tell you and responding therapeutically is now an accepted part of nursing care. The following article gives some easily understood guidelines that help us to evaluate our own skills while talking and listening to patients.

The habit of social conversation is ingrained in our culture. As a rule, such conversation is a give-and-take process

We went to Lake Tahoe for our vacation this year and . . . . Oh, you did! We flew to Hawaii for a week and had a wonderful time . . . . We took it easy for three weeks, fishing, hiking . . . .

The conversation shifts back and forth, focusing on no one particular contribution. But if we examine these statements the tendency toward "one upmanship" is obvious. The first person vacationed in Tahoe, the second flew to Hawaii for a week, but the first person had a three-week vacation.

One upmanship frequently occurs when two or three mothers talk about their children. Instead of actively listening, taking in, and understanding, the listener, instead, is contemplating the remarks he will make at the next pause!

The pleasant repartee of daily living has a definite and useful place in our culture. However, it also can be used to set the stage for truly therapeutic communication.

THERAPEUTIC COMMUNICATION

Fear and anxiety use up a patient's energy. The nurse who helps a patient to verbalize such feelings and bring them into the open can help him redirect his energies to the cause of establishing good health.

If encouraged, a patient may voice his reaction to his illness or his feelings about his dependency upon others. By openly expressing himself and explaining to another how he feels, a patient's fleeting, nebulous thoughts must, of necessity, become precise words and structured sentences.

Words and sentences require organization of thought processes which help a patient center his attention around a particular idea for a period of time. The physical act of speaking requires a close examination of thought. It requires more time to speak than to think, and thoughts are heard by the speaker himself.

Through the use of therapeutic communication, a nurse is able to clear the way for her patient to make his own decisions and to come to his own conclusions. How much more meaningful such determinations are for him than if they had been made by another "for his own good!"

NONDIRECTIVE TECHNIQUES

The use of some pleasantries or social intercourse is necessary to establishing an initial rapport and create a climate for more meaningful conversation. When common ground has thus been reached, the patient may begin to move the conversation toward an area of concern to him. Such an *opening statement* should be nonthreatening to the patient:

I see from the doctor's orders you are going home today, or You
appear anxious, or Dr. Jones says you are interested in breast-feeding
your baby, or You seem to be uncomfortable.

Such questions as, "Isn't it wonderful that you are going home today?" or "Why are you so anxious?" demand an answer, whereas a simple statement allows the patient a choice of continuing or not.

Once the broad opening statement has been made by nurse or patient, the next step is to keep the communication flowing. Several techniques can be employed to accomplish this.

The patient is encouraged to go on when he feels his remarks are accepted and not judged or evaluated by the listener. This can be done by nonverbal and/or verbal means. For example, a nod of the head or such comments by the nurse as "Uh-Huh!" "I see," "Yes."

Reflecting is another technique which keeps conversation flowing. The reflection may consist of a portion of the more significant points of a patient's cognitive dialogue as, for example.

Mrs. J: "I've had new pacemakers put in four times this year.

Nurse: Four times?

Mrs. J: Yes. The wire keeps slipping out and I'm getting so disgusted.

The nurse also can encourage the patient to explore feeling tones through the use of reflection. For example, continuing the above conversation . . .

Nurse: You're disgusted?

Mrs. J: Maybe that's not the word. I'm really afraid of where it is all going to end.

Her underlying fears becomes apparent.

Reflection gives feedback and essentially says, "Yes, I understand, you may continue if you wish." The questioning inflection in the nurse's voice asks, "Am I correct in what I understand you to say?"

The comment "Yes" by a patient only denotes that he believes the nurse has understood him correctly. However, a simple "yes" or "no" response to reflection may not necessarily be the end of a patient's reply to the statement.

Silence has advantages in therapeutic communication. A short pause after using reflection or other therapeutic techniques may encourage the patient to continue. He may need this time to consider what he has said and perhaps organize his thoughts for further communication. Silence also may be viewed as a kind of acceptance.

A nurse could well utilize this silent interval as an opportunity to formulate a response to her patient, instead of blurting out an immediate reaction. *Open ended phrases,* such as, "You were saying. . . ." "You want to go home because. . . ." "And then you. . . ." tend to encourage discussion by the patient in greater depth. Such phrases are particularly helpful when the conversation seems to be wandering away from the area of prime concern, or drifting into less meaningful communication. They also serve to emphasize to the patient that the nurse's interest in his concerns parallels his own.

The *use of the word "feeling"* when communicating often helps the patient to focus upon emotions rather than upon related factual information. For instance, "What are your feelings concerning your rehabilitation program?" or "How do you feel about going to a nursing home?" To be most effective, this technique requires a trusting relationship beyond just the initial rapport.

Summarizing a patient's dialogue is a method of mirroring his thoughts back to him. Thus, he may see himself, his attitudes, his opinions, and his plans in a clearer light. By pinpointing his most salient remarks, the nurse clarifies their meaning both to the patient and to herself. If a patient is speaking of a problem and its related conditions, the nurse can crystallize this information for him, thereby enhancing his capability of making his own decisions.

As with reflecting, summarizing gives the patient feedback, apprising him of the listener's comprehension as well as his own thoughts. Where, however, reflection is brief, a reiteration of only a few words or an attitude, summarizing reviews an entire idea or thought.

A summarizing statement may begin with "Do I understand you to say. . .?" "You seem to be saying that. . . ." "In other words you feel that. . ."

In addition to the spoken word, much human communication is carried on in a nonverbal fashion. Therapeutic verbal communication should be accompanied by actions which enhance the desired atmosphere. Expression, stance, and gestures, all combine to relate information to the observer and reinforce or even negate the spoken word.

A nurse can learn a great deal about a patient by observing his behavior. Conversely, the patient can learn much about a nurse's understanding and interest level through her mannerisms. Seated with chair close to patient, leaning forward, interested facial expressions, and frequent eye contact, will denote a feeling of empathy with the patient. Hands should be still for finger tapping and other nervous gestures will be interpreted as impatience.

Nondirective techniques, in addition to allowing the patient freedom to talk, help to keep the nurse from inadvertently making value statements and judgmental comments, common in everday conversation, which could easily be carried over to the patient-nurse interaction.

There is a tendency for nurses to respond with one of several clichés upon hearing of another's anxieties. "Don't worry. Everything is going to be all right." "Let's not talk about that just now." "You're lucky it wasn't worse." "Your doctor will take care of everything." "If you think you're bad off, look at the guy next to you."

Such remarks offer little solace to the patient and hinder further communication. Objectively considered, such clichés actually prove more soothing to the nurse than to the patient. Instead of conveying a message of comfort, they suggest, instead, an attitude of dismissal.

By relinquishing the automatic and stereotyped reactions of social communication, nurses can relate in more effective ways to patients. However, intellectual knowledge alone will not suffice. In order for communication techniques to be of value, they must be used, for it takes time and conscious effort to break old habits. But the self-discipline and energy required for this change become well worth the effort when a nurse receives the satisfaction of hearing a patient say, "Thanks for listening. Nobody else talks to me the way you do," or "I feel better, now."

Goldin and Russell suggest that the nurse make a nonthreatening statement to focus the conversation on the patient and his concerns. Dr. Peplau cautions against using two particular types of questions when attempting to help a patient focus on his needs. Write them here.

List at least two examples of a nonthreatening opening statement. Contrast these with a more threatening statement that demands answers.

Describe a nurse's posture or position that indicates understanding and interest in her patient while communicating.

List and describe, or give an example, of six nondirective techniques.

PATIENTS PROBLEM SOLVING

6.

Handicapped Patients Talk Together

Vera Heller

As you read this article, look at what fundamental information and skills this nursing student is applying. The explanation of the grief process was intentionally omitted from this article, since this subject is dealt with in greater depth in Part III.

During the last semester of my student nursing experience, much of my time was spent working with disabled patients on a newly established rehabilitation unit. It was not until then that I fully realized that physical restoration of a handicapped body cannot be separated from care of the whole patient—an essential concept of patient care in every field of nursing, In actually working with these patients I became more and more aware of the many avenues open for nursing intervention.

Expressions of feelings—anger, hostility, crying, fear, helplessness, and confusion—do not mean that these patients are uncooperative, stubborn, ornery, or ungrateful. Rather, these expressions are the normal, expected reactions to a difficult situation, created by the loss of body parts or functions. I recognized that although my patients were receiving good physical care, there was a lack of psychosocial care. Very little opportunity was provided for them to express their feelings, attitudes, and concerns.

I began to think of ways of changing this situation. I considered initiating group discussion among the patients, but, I was concerned about my lack of psychiatric expertise. Then I realized that informal group discussions, rather than psychotherapy, as such, might be an effective way to reach some of the patients. An informal setting for group discussion, I believed, might encourage a number of patients to get together to express and discuss their feelings and their concerns.

Before I presented my idea to the medical and nursing staffs for approval, I had to do two things. First, I needed to familiarize myself with the dynamics and processes of groups and, second, I needed to formulate definite objectives to substantiate my reasons for group discussions.

Next, I formulated more definite objectives:

1. To guide a selected number of patients for an hour, twice a week, in a group setting.

2. To establish an atmosphere which would be conducive to individual thought and increased self-awareness.

3. To provide an opportunity for emotional release through discussion and sharing of feelings, beliefs, and other attitudes regarding patients' physical disabilities.

4. To help patients, through this discussion and sharing, to find emotional support and understanding from each other and to acquire a feeling of belonging, thereby aiding them along their long and difficult road to adjustment.

5. To increase my leadership skills and to gain a deeper understanding of patients who are physically handicapped.

I received approval for my project from the head nurse, the area supervisor, the associate director of nursing, and the chief physician of the rehabilitation unit. The chief physician imposed one condition: that I have the supervision of a psychiatrist in the hospital's mental health department. The psychiatrist agreed to meet with me each week, and enthusiastically gave his approval. Then I requested support from the rest of the nursing staff on the unit. I hoped that through their participation at least one staff member would become interested enough to take over the group after I left, providing the group approach proved effective.

The head nurse helped me select prospective participants who had some physical disability, were not bedridden, and were able to communicate verbally. She also shared with me information regarding aspects of these patients' personal lives, behaviors, and likes or dislikes so that I could have background knowledge about each patient.

Before the first session, my anxiety level was sky-high. How should I begin? How should I deal with a long period of silence, should it occur? What should I do if some patients got angry and decided to leave? And, finally, in my state of anxiety, I began to doubt whether I really could lead a group by myself. I also anticipated that the patients were probably somewhat anxious, too, since, for the majority of them, it was a first experience in this type of a group setting.

THE FIRST MEETING

We were seated in a circle, and I made certain that the patients were physically as comfortable as possible. I introduced myself, explained the general purpose and objectives for the meetings, and their length and frequency. I also prepared them for the possibility of a changing membership, since some patients might be discharged from the hospital, while new patients might join us.

Then I suggested that each patient introduce himself to give each one an opportunity to say something and, at least superficially, get acquainted.

During that first session, feelings did emerge. Mr. S. introduced himself; he then continued.

Mr. S.: I could say something else too, but I better not! He looked around the room. Are there any tape-recorders or microphones?

Student: No, there are not. *(I had neglected to inform the patients of the confidentiality of the group's interactions.)*

Mr. S.: Well, it is about the nurses. They are always too busy to do anything for you. They never smile, just order you around, honey, sweetie, do such and such. They used to call me Pops, but I did not answer to that, so finally they remembered my name. There is only one nurse on the night shift who treats you as an adult human being!

Mrs. C.: Well, when I first came here I felt lost.

Student: You felt lost?

Mrs. C.: Yes, no one told me where anything was. I did not know who was what. They accused me of things I did not do, and they threatened me by saying that if I pushed the buzzer once more, it would be a long time before anybody answered my bell.

Several patients expressed similar negative experiences, until Mrs. J. spoke.

Mrs. J.: For myself, I like it here. For most of my life I have had to cater to other people, but now I can relax, sleep, get clean sheets and bedclothes every day, and get my meals served to me. I never had that before.

When I announced that it was time to end the session Mr. S. raised a question.

Mr. S.: What is the use of complaining? This was just a bull session, what good does it do?

Mr. K.: At least you got it off your chest and that is better than keeping it inside.

Student: Often we have to express those feelings that are closest to the surface and that concern us most at the moment before we are able to discuss anything else.

Even though the main theme of this discussion was patients' expressions about the nursing care they had received, rather than their own feelings and perceptions of self, I thought the session was of value. Perhaps because the discussion was based on the common ground of hospitalization, the patients seemed relaxed and were spontaneous in their interactions.

Two patients refused to come back for the second group meeting. Even though I knew I should have expected this, I felt that I had failed in some way. I tried to reconstruct the first session, hoping that I would find a reason, either in the group process or in my own conduct, which could have been responsible for the patients' refusals. The patients stated several reasons. However, the message they seemed to convey to me was that they felt uncomfortable in a group setting, thought they might not be accepted by the others, or were afraid of revealing too much of themselves.

During my first consultation with the psychiatrist, I expressed my concern about the refusal of the two patients to continue in the group. After reviewing with him the topics we had discussed and the interactions, that had taken place, Dr. W. said that it was to be expected that several patients would refuse to continue in a group. He suggested that I make a more definite verbal contract with the patients and that perhaps the most appropriate way for me to lead this group was to observe the patients' actions, and reflect on their comments and nonverbal communications.

Five patients participated in the second group meeting. One patient had been discharged, but Mrs. H., a new patient, joined us. The topics discussed dealt with the patients' feelings about their dependent state and about death.

Mr. H.: The most important thing to me is to get back on my feet and be able to get around by myself. I have always been independent and am used to doing everything for myself.

Mrs. H.: That is how I feel. I want to get back on my feet and go home. I hate to have to ask for every little thing that I always used to do for myself.

The other patients nodded in agreement, except for Mrs. M., who seemed to function best when she was dependent on someone else.

The rest of the time was spent on the issue of death. It was brought up by Mr. S., who said that death could be a blessing for some people who suffer from incurable, progressively debilitating illnesses.

Mrs. J.: The one thing we own in life is death. We all die but the Lord guaranteed us eternal life.

Mr. K.: I must disagree with you. Death owns us. When it comes, it does, and there is no power in this world that can prevent it. (I believe he was referring to the sudden death of his 12-year-old daughter, during which time he suffered a cerebral vascular accident.)

Mrs. M.: I know we must all die, but I do not want to die yet; there are still things that I want to do when I get well.

Another patient was discharged; thus, the number of participants in the group decreased to four. During the third session, patients expressed feelings regarding fear of their illnesses, the implications, and their feelings of helplessness. For example:

Mr. H.: When I get those cramps I feel like dying. There can't be anything worse. I am scared, just plain scared, waiting for the next attack. I am scared of the unknown. I wonder what part of me will become paralyzed next. They will not let me take the pills at my own discretion; they are afraid I will commit suicide.

Mr. K.: You need more than one pill to commit suicide. The truth is that one does feel frightened. Here you are lying in bed, knowing quite well that if you need something or if something happens, there is nothing you can do about it, except to wait and hope that someone will come to your aid.

Student: Is what you are expressing perhaps a feeling of helplessness?

Mr. K.: Yes! To know that you cannot do the things that you used to is bad enough, but to feel helpless is even worse.

After this session, I realized that I no longer was experiencing feelings of anxiety; I was relaxed, and more confident in my ability as a leader of a group. The group was progressing from more general topics to expressions of more individual feelings. This became even more evident during the next session.

Mr. H.: Last night I woke up and wanted to put my left hand on my chest but I couldn't find it! Then I realized that it was on my chest all this time. It sure scared me.

Mr. K.: You too? The same thing happens to me; sometimes I cannot really feel the left side of my body. It is like a dead weight. It makes me feel as if I am only half a man.

Mrs. R.: I know what you mean. (Tears in her eyes) I can't do anything with my hands. Hands are so important. You do everything with them. I can't even clean the house, cook, or even feed myself.

The focus of the fifth meeting was interests, hobbies, and goals before their illnesses. I thought the group, perhaps, was regressing, that the patients were trying to divert the discussion from their own problems to a more comfortable topic. However, during my consultation with the psychiatrist, Dr. W. explained that discussing one's hobbies, interests, and goals was talking about one's self, although in an indirect and safer way. He also explained that interests and hobbies can reflect personality.

As each person talked about his interests, I could see that Dr. W. was right. Mr. H., still a big, robust man, talked about his interest in baseball and football. Mrs. R. talked about her interest in cooking and handwork. These were hobbies and interests that could not now be pursued by these patients due to their physical disabilities. Perhaps they were really expressing grief about what they were missing.

THE LAST MEETINGS

Before the end of the session, I reminded the patients that I would soon be leaving, but that Mrs. McC., the occupational therapist, would like to come to our next meeting, and perhaps take over when I left. I asked the patients if they had any objections. There was a moment of silence but, then, they all gave their consent. I had previously discussed this with Dr. W. At first, he seemed concerned with the difficulty the occupational therapist and the patients might have in adjusting to the new role she would have to assume as a group leader while still an occupational therapist to these patients. However, we agreed that since she was interested in the continuation of the group, patients would benefit more if the group were continued than if it ended when I left.

Mrs. McC. joined us during the next group discussion. I noticed that the patients, at first, were somewhat reluctant to start the discussion. However, after initial introductions, they continued the previous week's topic of discussion and further shared their feelings and concerns. One important interaction occurred:

Mrs. M.: (to Mr. H.) How did you get injured?

Mr. H.: I was born with a bad spine but that is not my problem now. I first began to realize that there was something wrong when my left foot started swinging outward. For years, the doctors thought I had arthritis. You always read that they are close to the cure of arthritis. Then things got worse, and they told me that I didn't have arthritis, but, rather, progressive paralysis which can't be cured.

Mrs. R.: It must have been very difficult for you to learn that.

Mr. K.: It sure was. After I got my hopes up about being cured, I found out that I had something for which there is no cure.

Mr. K.: It must have been very disappointing and discouraging for you.

There was very little need for me to interject anything. These patients were supporting each other.

After the session ended, Mrs. R. told me that she was glad she had joined us because she felt that it was good for her to talk about her problems. Mr. H. told me he thought he would never have wanted to be in a group like this.

My objectives for this project were accomplished to some degree.

During the last three meetings several things began to happen. The group seemed to gain more cohesiveness and unity. The patients seemed to identify more as members of the group. They began to realize that their problems and difficulties were not isolated but, rather, were shared by other members. Their original preoccupation with individual problems seemed to become somewhat replaced by mutual understanding and support. There was also increasing self-awareness.

I increased my skill in leadership and gained a much deeper understanding of the difficulties and problems that physically handicapped patients face. I also realized that students of nursing can initiate and carry out some aspects of total patient care not done before.

Which of the following skills did Miss Heller need to use in her group work with patients?

Awareness of anxiety in one's self and others.

Use of nondirective techniques.

Leading a group discussion.

Observing behavior.

Recognizing when feelings are being expressed.

Knowing how to ask for help from experts or resource people.

Working with other members of the health team.

Initiating, maintaining, and terminating a relationship.

When looking over this list an outsider might ask, "But why is this important in order to nurse a patient?" How would you reply?

How do you view health and illness? Optimum functioning? How is this nursing student helping these patients return to optimum functioning?

Does this nursing role differ from the roles of the other members on the health team? If so, how and why?

Describe the steps Miss Heller took to overcome her anxiety as she prepared to initiate the group discussion.

7.
Communication Through Role Playing

Patricia R. Underwood

Why do you use role playing? How does it help your communication skills? This article describes how patients can be helped with their communication skills in much the same way that you are. Another way to "nurse" patients!

Role playing might best be defined as a learning experience in which the nurse and the patient act out a situation, either past or expected, as if it were really happening. They might act out a discussion the patient has already had with a family member or a job interview the patient is anticipating. The situation to be acted out depends on the needs of the patient. I found it valuable in working with Mary.

Mary was a 20-year-old, unskilled factory worker with nine years of education, a history of immature acting-out behavior, and limited communication with her family. She had immigrated to the United States 11 years ago.

I saw Mary shortly after her admission to a residential home for unwed mothers, angry, frightened, unable to adjust to the residential center. After several meetings with her, I found she thought there was something wrong with her or her unborn baby. Our discussion revealed an underlying fear of doctors and nurses based on a few unhappy encounters. She was unable to ask questions of the doctor or nurse and left each antepartal examination frightened and certain she was ill. To help her overcome her fears, I tried role playing.

Mary: I have an itch down here. (She indicated the pubic area.)

Nurse: That is something the doctor should know.

Mary: You know I can't tell him.

Nurse: Let's try. I'll be the doctor and you be you. O.K., tell me.

Mary: I have an itch down here. (She laughs and blushes.) That sounds funny. What do you call this?

Nurse: It's the pubic area.

Mary: I have an itch in—on—which is it? (laughs)

Nurse: Try "around."

Mary: I have an itch around the pubic area.

Doctor (as played by the nurse): How long have you had it?

Mary (relaxing): About two weeks.

Doctor: Can you show me exactly where it is?

Mary: Right here.

Nurse: Good, that's it. You'll be able to talk to the doctor and tell him how you feel.

Mary had numerous other questions about her pregnancy that had been on her mind for weeks, questions that could easily have been answered by the nurse. But role playing with less complicated questions helped her to learn to express herself more directly. Over the weeks we worked on more difficult areas until she was able to talk to the doctor with ease. Her sense of well-being increased as her self-confidence increased, and this encouraged her to try talking more directly not only with me and the physician, but also with other staff members and with patients in the residence.

Mary had difficulty in communicating with her family and rarely disagreed or openly resisted decisions they made. She simply did not comply with decisions she did not like. That usually got her into trouble. Although she did not really want to relinquish her child, Mary agreed with her family's decision that she should. She said her family made her depressed. Believing they did not understand her, she felt angry and resentful toward her family. However, she did not recognize the anger she felt. Again role playing helped.

Mary: I wish they would quit asking about what I'm going to do and then saying what I have to do.

Nurse: That must make you angry.

Mary: No! I just feel low.

Nurse: What do you do when they start telling you?

Mary: Nothing; just listen.

Nurse: What would you like to do?

Mary: I don't know.

Nurse: Let's role play. I'll be your brother Joe and you be you. (I had seen the brother once, and Mary had talked about him quite often. Even if the nurse doesn't know the person she is playing, the situation will build as one gets into it.)

Joe: Well, Mary, what have you decided? Have you seen the adoption lady? You should begin to plan.

Mary: Just shut up! I don't want to plan anything. I don't know what to do.

Joe: Why are you yelling at me? I asked you a simple question.

Mary: Nag, nag, nag. That's all you ever do. I hate you and I'm tired of it all. (The patient looked at me bewildered.) What did I say?

Nurse: You seemed to be saying what you felt. You're pretty upset with your brother who is pushing you.

Mary: But I don't hate him. He has been good to me.

Nurse: It's all right to be angry. You can love and hate at the same time.

Mary: I shouldn't have said that.

Nurse: It was the way you were feeling.

Mary: But that would just make him mad at me.

Nurse: What might you say that would get the point across without making him angry? I'll be Joe again.

Joe: Well, what are you going to do? You should be thinking about what to do with the baby.

Mary: (looking straight at me, speaking with a calm, confident voice): I don't know. I haven't decided. When I do, I will tell you.

Joe: O.K., Mary. As long as you're thinking about it.

Nurse: That's it. There is nothing left to say. Now you be your brother, and I'll be you, Mary.

We exchanged roles and repeated that conversation. Mary had the same feeling I had had: She had made a final statement that left no room for further questioning. Mary then used this approach with her brother. He responded by telling her to let him know what she decided. He did not question her further. Shortly thereafter, Mary was able to begin to work on her feelings about the child she was expecting and to decide what she was going to do.

We used role playing to clarify her feelings regarding what to say if she met someone who was a patient with her in the residence; what to say if Aunt Sally remarked that she was fat; how to tell her mother that she wanted to use contraceptives, and how to ask the doctor for contraceptives; how to obtain information about enrolling in a school of beauty culture rather than returning to the factory to work.

When the baby was about seven days overdue, Mary began to feel helpless and depressed. She cried, was despondent and unable to talk about her feelings. Her anger seemed to be directed toward the baby and herself. She berated the unborn child and would then feel guilty and still more depressed. I tried a different version of role playing.

Mary (looking at her abdomen): You stupid thing. Why don't you come out? I hate you. You are seven days late, and you just sit there.

Nurse: If the baby could talk to you, what would he say?

Mary (after some hesitation, surprised at the question, responding in an angry voice): It's not my fault. I didn't put me here; you did. I don't know why you yell at me. I'd like to get out too.

Nurse: The baby seems angry too.

Mary: Why shouldn't he be. He's right! I put him there. It's all my fault. God is punishing me.

That allowed the whole area of punishment to surface, and Mary could talk about fears previously expressed only in tears and berating of the baby. She could recognize that the anger she felt was actually toward herself rather than the child. She was able to verbalize rather than internalize her anger.

The foregoing are only a few examples of how effective role playing can be. It allowed me to utilize rather than overlook basic differences—in this instance socioeconomic differences. I could work at the educational level of the patient without embarrassing her. On the other hand, Mary got immediate satisfaction, quick results. Role playing added action to the interview sessions, and Mary felt she was getting something done, not "just talking." And it opened areas that might otherwise have remained closed to both the nurse and the patient.

As with any other interpersonal technique, role playing is not appropriate for every situation. It can, however, be a very simple and effective tool for improving communications, understanding, and treatment.

How do you imagine the nurse found out that the patient was afraid that something was wrong with her unborn baby and that she had a fear of nurses and doctors? What did she do to get this information?

What future health problems might be averted because of the patient's improved ability to communicate?

Where else might such a situation occur other than in a home for unwed mothers? Where can the nurse practice preventive nursing?

8.

It's the Patient's Problem — and Decision

Karyl K. Blair

*You have read that therapeutic communication helps a patient
increase his capacity to make his own decisions. The following
article describes how this strength is not only talked about but
put into practice. This article is concerned with how a public
health nursing staff changed their approach to patient care and
found that patients could better use their own strengths when the
nurses allowed them an active role in attaining their own goals.
The implications to be found in their story are unlimited.*

*Whether caring for patients in the home, hospital, office or some
other health facility, we always need to be aware of how our
actions affect the recipients of our care. Are we making our
patients docile and dependent in order to keep things going on
schedule or are we challenging their inner free spirits to emerge and
assert themselves? Are we willing to accept patients' rights to
reject care and ourselves at times? It is hard to give up control
when you are accustomed to being an authority figure but the
results seen in this article may convince you to try.*

The public health nursing agency with which I am connected has, over the past
two years, not only changed its approach to the patients it serves and developed
a new way of working with them, but it has also reevaluated its whole
philosophy for providing health care services. The new philosophy has meant

that, in effect, we have rejected the usual concept of "total patient care" by the nurse that we learned in school and have replaced it with one that encourages the patient to act for himself.

This quite dramatic change was the result of an experience in psychiatric consultation that started at a time when the morale of our agency had hit a low point. We were unable to perform many of the activities considered necessary for providing total patient care. Requests for service were accumulating on our desks, while, at the same time, the staff were making five to seven home visits a day that often required 50 to 100 miles of driving. We had no time to meet requests for consultation with other groups, such as schools.

A NEW WAY OF HELPING OTHERS

When our nursing agency reached its lowest ebb, with the resignation of the senior nurse, our entire staff began to meet with the consulting psychiatrist who had been hired for the new community program. His main requirement for the use of his time was that we discuss a specific family situation about which the concerned nurse had written a summary of the problem and the help she wanted prior to the consultation session. Thus, we focused on specific questions and problems which made the application of the consultant's help quite obvious. Every other week for an hour and a half we discussed with him the families with whom we were having problems—not necessarily families with diagnosed mental illness—and from this experience we learned a whole new way of helping others.

At first, though, we used our time to discuss those families in which one member had a diagnosed mental illness; often, someone who had been discharged from the state mental hospital. At a consultation session that is memorable to me, we discussed my biggest challenge at that time—a woman with a diagnosis of chronic paranoid schizophrenia, who had a history of several hospitalizations. Since she was verbalizing her psychotic thinking fairly freely at that time, my plan called for seeing her weekly—at least trying to, for often she would not answer the door—in order to develop a closer relationship with her so she could. . . .Well, somehow, that was supposed to make her better.

At this session, as the psychiatrist discussed the behavior of this patient with me, he began to ask questions. "What is the purpose of your visits? Why are you seeing her every week? Why do you need to stay for an hour? Does the patient want you to come? What are the patient's goals?" My mental rebuttal was, "This patient has problems. Isn't it obvious that she needs me?"

TREATMENT SHORTCOMINGS

As a result of the consultation and discussion in relation to this patient, as well as of many other patients, the staff began to recognize certain shortcomings in our treatment plans. We learned, for instance, that there is sometimes danger in letting a patient express too many feelings. We came to understand that lengthy sessions with patients are not only inefficient ways of dealing with their behavior problems, but are also often harmful to them; and we also learned the supportive value of seeing a psychotic patient for not more than 15 to 20 minutes once a month.

Frequently, the nurse can be destructive to a person's self-esteem through her well-meaning, subtle efforts to increase a patient's insight. We have learned the value of focusing the patient's thinking and comments on reality events, rather than letting him live in the past or in his fantasy life through verbalization.

ESTABLISHING A CONTRACT

During these two years of psychiatric consultation, we have discussed a variety of families from among our cases. Usually the family has been one with a behavior pattern that is interfering with its ability to find answers to its health problems. The emphasis has been on the patient and his family. Increasingly, the key question has become: what is the patient asking for? It is surprising how much the answering of this question helps the nurse understand many other things, including where she should start, how clearly the patient sees his problem, and whether or not the nurse should even be in the home.

We have learned the importance of establishing a contract with the patient—that is, a mutual understanding of the reason for the service and the problems or areas that will be discussed during the visits. This contract results from the nurse's discussion and clarification with the patient as to what he actually wants and what services she can provide. In establishing a contract, we have found it most helpful to set a specified limit—either in length of time to be expended or in a given number of visits. Then the contract is reviewed for possible extension, renegotiation, or termination.

In addition to establishing this understanding with each patient, we have developed a firm commitment to the philosophy of promoting the patient's strengths. It is imperative that the patient recognize and use his own strengths to solve his own problems. One can observe a family, a staff, or an administrator in many ways, which could fall on a continuum from very negative to very positive.

It is obvious that one cannot use what doesn't exist, but there is a tendency to concentrate on what one does not have or, in this case, what the patient cannot do; that is, to emphasize the negative. For example, Mrs. Smith cannot toilet-train her child; family X has no insurance for medical care; Susie will not wear her hearing aid; Grandma Jones refuses to do her range of motion exercises; or Mrs. Y will not follow her diabetic diet.

A nurse's encounter with a patient is usually generated by a crisis of greater or lesser magnitude. For a patient to rally and gain from the crisis, he needs to recognize his strengths in terms of what *does* exist. Every home has some positive aspect, whether it is a bouquet of lilacs on the table, a new piece of furniture, or a warm relationship among family members. It is surprising how many patients and families can gain energy from having someone point out existing strengths. With this added energy, they are able to make plans for solving their own health problems.

EMPHASIS ON STRENGTHS

Another key element in this approach, a corollary to focusing on patient strengths, has been the emphasis on patient autonomy. What actually can the patient do for himself? Patients *can* make telephone calls themselves to obtain information. They *do* find suitable answers to health problems, sometimes without any nursing assistance. More important, patients *do* have the right to accept or reject our service. When a patient is allowed to carry out his decision, he feels like a respectable person with some degree of wellness. When we expect our patients to initiate action of their own, we further promote wellness. The more often the patient is told, explicitly or implicitly, that he has a degree of wellness because he can do some things for himself, the more he progresses.

On careful reflection, I think that what we have really changed in our program is our concept of "total patient care." I feel strongly that this term—total patient care—has connotations that are not only far beyond the realm of reality, but also are destructive to the patient. It implies, at least to many new graduates, that the patient is completely helpless and that the nurse must do everything (total care) for him. The nurse thus accepts responsibility for solving the patient's problem rather than crediting him with the ability to find his own solution with or without her assistance.

Our staff can now accept the fact that the patient himself must make the decisions about his care. In fact, we feel that nursing service will be helpful only *if* the patient has made decisions about his plan of care. We can help him implement his plan, but he can elect to follow a plan that does not seem appropriate to us.

The positive result is that the patient no longer needs to use his energy to think of ways of staying out of reach of the persistent nurse; he can use it for problem-solving and for healing.

Because the nurse does not feel a need to hold the patient to her concept of a solution, she does not feel she has failed if her solutions or expectations do not seem appropriate to the patient. Thus, she is able to let the patient solve more of his problems. As a result, we have seen many almost miraculous changes in the families with whom we work.

The psychotic patient mentioned earlier, for instance, remains at home, and her level of functioning continues to improve. When, after the psychiatric consultation pertaining to her case, I asked her how she felt about the frequency of home visits, her look of shock and disbelief was followed by, "Come however often you're supposed to come." She communicated the feeling of being in the tight vicelike grip of the professionals who were treating her like a puppet. This feeling only created anxiety for her ("What will they make me do next?"), resulting in her escape to psychotic thinking and verbalization. Together, we agreed on monthly visits of from 15 to 45 minutes, which she has not avoided for nine months.

This specific contract, combined with support of her ideas and recognition of her accomplishments in the home, has been rewarded by her more appropriate behavior. She now takes some responsibility for housekeeping tasks; she is using her sewing machine; she stays on her medications; she stays off her beer; and she talks directly to her husband and children. Last week, she mentioned a desire to look into the possibility of obtaining the equivalent of a high school diploma. There are indications that specific plans for termination of nursing service will soon be discussed.

What was the key question that guided the planning of their nursing care? How might you establish a contract with a patient that you were going to help regain bowel control? What patient strengths would you look for and discuss with the patient? Why should you make a point to discuss his strengths before stating what you, the nurse, have to offer? What would you do if the patient rejected your offer of help?

Think of other patient situations where you and the patient need to work together to improve his level of health. Ask yourself these same questions with each patient example until you begin to see the value of this approach.

9.

Can Nursing Care Hasten Recovery?

Cynthia Henderson

Nursing care – what do you think of when you hear this term? Who gives "nursing care" in your community? Think of the purpose of nursing care and the reasons for having an R.N. give this care. The following article will show you how nurses put into practice their theory regarding the importance of patients making decisions and of nurses observing and communicating.

Look for the criteria for admissions to the nursing care center described below. How do these differ from admissions in a general hospital? Look for the difference in job descriptions of auxiliary personnel. How does this differ from the roles of R.N.s, L.P.N.s, nurse's aides and unit secretaries in your community agency?

There *is* something new under the sun—a center for nursing! Not a medical, not a psychiatric, not a day-care, or geriatric, or maternity, or recreation, or research center, but the 80-bed Loeb nursing center which is dedicated to the belief that around-the-clock care by registered nurses will help sick people heal faster.

Loeb eludes cataloguing as an institution principally because it cares for those patients who no longer need the intensive medical diagnostic and therapeutic measures—the crisis-therapy, if you will—for which most patients are presently admitted to hospitals. Loeb accepts the patient from the hospital after extensive work-up is complete, his surgery performed, or his medical treatment under way, at a point of illness during which he still requires medical supervision, but of an evaluative nature. Also, and herein lies this center's individuality, Loeb accepts a patient at that time when professional nursing care can help him enter into the healing process.

A halfway house on the road home for persons who have had congestive heart failure, a colostomy, a badly fractured femur, or an enucleation, Loeb intends not to duplicate any other facility. A patient with quadriplegia, for example, requires prolonged intensive rehabilitation which he can best receive at a rehabilitation center. The psychotic individual will improve faster in a setting equipped to offer daily therapy in the protective atmosphere which only the psychiatric agency provides. Loeb seeks those hospitalized persons in need, primarily, of the teaching, counseling, and nurturing which are inherent in professional nursing.

Loeb's administrative director, Lydia Hall; the medical consultant, Dr. Harold Rifkin; and a social worker screen applicants for admission by these criteria: Will this person benefit from intensive professional nursing care? Has he a reasonable chance of returning to the community within a prescribed time? Is his stage of illness such that he can become actively involved in working through problems of regaining health?

If the answers are "yes", and the applicant is at least 16 years old, he is transferred from Montefiore, or any other acute hospital, to the open and more homelike nursing center. Diagnosis is less a determinant for admission than stage of illness.

Loeb Center's most distinctive feature is that all direct patient care is given by registered nurses. The staff of 35 full-time professional nurses includes five senior staff positions which require at least a baccalaureate degree, one chief nurse, an assistant director, and a director. Besides these, there are two regular part-time registered nurses and a few who work occasionally on a per diem basis. The ratio is one registered nurse to each eight patients and their families during both day and evening hours. At night, the ratio widens on the assumption that a patient who has had intensive professional care for 16 hours will sleep.

THE VITAL DIFFERENCE

There are no practical nurses or aides at Loeb because Lydia Hall believes that it is the professional nurse, with her background in biological, physical, and social sciences, who is most able to give the intimate bodily care—bathing, feeding, toileting, dressing, positioning, and moving and best prepared to use the closeness of this relationship to help a patient regain his health. If the professional nurse delegates this core of nursing's exclusive body of knowledge to less-prepared personnel, the patient loses the support of the one person most qualified to work with him, she maintains.

Each staff nurse is assigned a block of eight rooms; she works with patients from their admission until discharge. Length of hospital stay during Loeb's first year of operation has varied from two weeks to six months, with an average of about 30 days.

Secretaries do the telephone and paper work, limited as compared to that in the acute hospital since Loeb's patients are beyond the busy diagnostic testing phase. To run errands, to bring equipment, to provide a nurse with the "things" essential to her care at the bedside, one messenger-attendant is employed for each two registered nurses. Whatever is done directly with the patient is done by the professional nurse.

For instance, the nurse helps toilet patients because it is during elimination that a patient is most apt to express concern about bowel problems. Originally, the nurses felt that they should also empty bedpans. But as they analyzed *when* the patient might voice his problems, they realized that it often was in those few minutes while the nurse was away taking care of equipment. Therefore, emptying pans became a messenger-attendant's task.

The messenger-attendants are employed without previous hospital background so that they will not expect to give direct care. Staff nurses train them on the job and the lack of turnover among messenger-attendants indicates their enjoyment.

Messenger-attendants deliver and remove food trays. But if a patient's eyes are patched or his hands bandaged, it is the professional nurse who assists him to eat. Again, the closeness at mealtime offers natural opportunities for nurse and patient to work together.

OPEN ATMOSPHERE

Nursing *with* the patient is the core of Loeb's philosophy. In nearly every way conceivable, the place, the people, and the activities say, "We are with you." The two-story building has broad, pleasant corridors, wide doors to accommodate wheel chairs, cheerful day-recreation-dining rooms with access to the out of doors, attractive patient rooms which are decorated with taste and cheer, but not with such strident cheer that they upset a depressed patient. Nothing is locked except the medicine cabinets.

Loeb's "open" atmosphere includes its medical record in the sense that this has no order sheets by which physicians order nurses to order patients to do this or take that. Medical care plans are arrived at jointly by the doctors, nurses, and, to a considerable extent, the patients.

A newly admitted patient is not handed pills at arbitrarily prescribed times. Instead, the nurse first reviews with him any pharmacologic limits such as long or short action, or irritation to an empty stomach, then asks when he prefers his medicine, and she gives it at the hours he chooses. Usually, he tends gradually toward a balanced schedule.

Patient progress observations are written chronologically by every nurse and specialist. Physicians' comments are underlined in red for easy identification by house doctors pressed for time in emergency calls. Nursing observations include few, if any, statements of tasks performed, but many discussions of patient concerns, expressed verbally or by behavior, and nurses' responses. Dr. Rifkin cited as excellent, objective evidence of a man's ability to withstand emotional stress, this note by his evening nurse: "Had a heated argument with his roommate for 10 or 15 minutes. This did not seem to affect his color or breathing in any way or cause him pain." The patient had both a ventricular aneurysm and a recent myocardial infarction.

Patients are encouraged to keep logs. Though these cannot, legally, be filed with the chart, a patient may share his log with his nurse or doctor. Even when he keeps it to himself, by writing out his feelings, he often identifies where he is and where he wants to go in the business of recovering.

One of his choices is the time he wishes to bathe. A patient just transferred from a hospital is apt to say, "Oh, I always take my bath in the morning." His nurse replies, "Fine, if you really like it then, but you may bathe at night." Conditioned by days or weeks of hospitalization to accomplish as much as possible between 7:00 A.M. and 3:30 P.M., he continues the morning bath. After a few days, as he sees his roommate helped into the shower by the evening nurse, and since he is still offered a choice—or even a second bath—he remembers that he always bathed at night and he switches.

FREE CHOICES

To quiet a wakeful patient at night the nurse tries tactfully to discover the reason for his insomnia. Perhaps he's hot or uncomfortable from lying too long in one position. Occasionally, analgesia or sedation is the answer; often the cause is loneliness or worry. Sometimes the nurse spends an hour or two listening, talking, reflecting with a sleepless patient. When finally he relaxes into sleep, she records her observations on his progress sheet which she and his day nurse will read together. He will not be awakened at the crack of dawn. Routines, such as temperature taking at 8:00-12:00-4:00-8:00, or everybody washed before 7:00 A.M., are rare at Loeb. Vital signs are taken once, at a time convenient to patient and nurse, during the late afternoon. Naturally, more frequent checking is done if the patient's illness warrants this.

Permissiveness extends to eating, both the where and the when. One woman recovering from radical gastric surgery said, "The best thing about Loeb is, if I wake up in the middle of the night with my stomach gnawing my backbone, the nurse will get anything I want to eat. . . . I sleep better after eating."

Patients decide where they will eat. Some, with handicaps which make them unattractive meal companions, prefer to be alone. ·

Families and friends, including children, may visit at any time, day or night.

When problems arise, as they inevitably do, because one patient in a two-bed room wishes to retire at 10:00 P.M. and his roommate's callers linger, the nurse works with each patient to help him see the other's point of view. Each 20-bed wing has a comfortable lounge where a parent may see his youngsters, or late visitors may talk without disturbing others. Visitors are encouraged and nurses work with patients' families.

Freedom of choice is not only a patient's prerogative. The staff may decide how to dress for duty. Many start out in uniform, eventually change to street clothes. Cotton blouses, full skirts, and duty shoes, or some variation, appear to be most popular. One nurse always wears her uniform because she "worked too hard for this cap and its stripe to give it up." For close bedside nursing, most of the staff don a full-length white apron. Patients' reactions to the absence of uniforms differ. One gentleman said, "Well, since I *am* a man, I like to see the girls dressed up instead of all in stiff white." A young woman disagreed, "There's nothing so dignified as a white uniform. Those white stockings—and that cap—they just *make* a nurse!"

"Do the nurses who wear uniforms give you better care?"

"Oh, no! A uniform doesn't make any difference about *that!*"

EMERGING TRENDS

Although 14 months' operation is too short a time in which to accumulate statistical proof of costs, bed utilization, or average length of admission, a few hours at Loeb Center prove it to be an exciting, growing, going concern. Certain trends emerge from a random sampling of responses to Loeb's follow-up questionnaires sent to physicians and patients after patients go home. Of 40 physician replies to the question, "By how many days was hospital stay shortened by use of Loeb Center?," the lowest answer was three days; the highest was 43 days; most doctors estimated that Loeb admission had shortened hospitalization by one to three weeks.

These 40 doctor replies to the query about the quality of nursing care (choices offered ranged from poor to excellent) included 1 "good", 38 "excellent", and 1 "superb." Patient reactions came, almost 100 percent, in superlatives—"wonderful," "out of this world," "only at Loeb could I have had care like this."

Adverse comments mentioned difficulty in identifying nurses because of lack of uniform, "food o.k., but not cooked the way I like it"; a physician expressed annoyance because he had not been notified that his patient had decided to prolong her stay by three days.

Some physicians have remarked that their patients not only recover faster, but maintain their gains after discharge. Others are watchfully studying what happens at Loeb, not yet wholly convinced. One cardiologist, somewhat dubious about the merits of a nursing center, transferred his first patient with myocardial infarction after her fourth week of hospitalization. She was ready for discharge in two weeks. Presently, this doctor transferred a patient with similar diagnosis at three weeks; the next at two. Both patients went home in two weeks. Now the doctor plans to move a patient to Loeb ten days after her infarction, and expects that she, too, will go home in two weeks.

Both Lydia Hall and Dr. Rifkin emphasize that these and other facts are indicative and encouraging, but not conclusive. However, Dr. Rifkin says, "I believe this kind of facility is the coming thing. I'd like to see a Loeb Center attached to every medical center, or better yet, I'd like to see Loeb's kind of nursing incorporated into every hospital."

Will Loeb reduce the cost of hospitalization to the patient? It is estimated that, when it is running at its 80-bed capacity, the rates will vary from $19 to $30 per day. The Department of Hospitals pays $17 per day toward costs of indigent patients. Peak census has been 67; at present it averages 44-48 not due to a shortage of applicants or staff, but because Loeb's experimental Blue Cross contract covered only the first 250 admissions. The 250 mark was reached far sooner than anyone had anticipated. A new contract is being negotiated, and early, full occupancy of the Loeb Center is expected.

The criticism has been made that Loeb's admission policies are highly selective. They must be, say both its director and its medical consultant, if Loeb is to test the theories it was built to evaluate. Without selectivity they say, Loeb would soon have a static population and become a custodial institution rather than a center for helping people who have a reasonable chance to return to the community.

An outsider takes away from Loeb many impressions: patients who enjoy their surroundings, understand their care, and praise their entertainment programs; physicians pleased, on the whole; nurses attracted to the center because they hope to practice as they were taught, staying because the hope is realized—and enlarged since this is bedside nursing in a much expanded manner.

Would you consider this team nursing? Why or why not?

What is the rationale for keeping the registered nurse at the bedside with the patient? Would this be considered "preventive nursing"?

Describe the atmosphere that is cultivated at Loeb Center. What are the areas in which patients are allowed to make choices about their nursing care?

How would this affect the routines and schedules in your community hospital? Which of the characteristics could be applied in your hospital?

This kind of nursing care is still in operation at Loeb. For further information you can write . . . . Miss Genrose Alfano, Director, Loeb Center for Nursing and Rehabilitation at Montefiore Hospital, Steuben Avenue and 210th Street, Bronx, New York.

PATIENT SITUATIONS

10.
When Adult Patients Cry

Gertrud B. Ujhely

Before reading the next article think about the last time you saw someone cry – preferably a stranger – what words would you use to describe your feelings? Write them here.

Now try to recall an instance of when you were crying in public when there were strangers or casual acquaintances around. Describe in writing how you felt in that situation and what you did when the urge or the actual crying occurred.

Think about what people around you did or how they reacted to your crying. Was it helpful or not and why?

After that bit of introspection you are ready to read the article. While reading, you may wish to compare your answers above with those in the article.

Among the patients whom many nurses consider "problem" patients are those who are in the process of losing control over their emotions. Examples of these are patients under the influence of alcohol; patients who, seemingly without prior provocation, become abusive or assaultive; patients who laugh inappropriately, and also patients who break down and cry.

From "When Adult Patients Cry" by Gertrud B. Ujhely, published in the December 1967 issue of Nursing Clinics of North America. *Copyright © December 1967 by the W. B. Saunders Company. Reproduced, with permission, from* Nursing Clinics of North America.

When asked what it is that makes these patients seem so difficult, nurses tend to say that they "dislike" them, that they are "uncomfortable" with them, or that they are at a loss as to "how to handle" them.

This is quite understandable, for we are not used to being confronted by raw emotionality. It is not acceptable in any culture to relate to others directly via our naked selves, as it were.

No wonder, then, that we become frightened if we see another's armor cracking or even disintegrating in front of our eyes. For what guarantee do we have that our own armor is going to hold up under the onslaught of this uncivilized behavior, especially when it is bombarded from the inside by our own emotions? Holding these in check is not an easy task for any nurse who is confronted every minute of her working day by human suffering and pain. And how are we to perform our necessary tasks if we, in turn, become flooded with our own emotions? It is not surprising, then, that nurses may consider the patient who is losing control of himself as a problem patient.

This paper will restrict itself only to one kind of patient in this group, namely the crying (or weeping) adult patient. It is anticipated, however, that it will be possible for the reader to make some inferences from what is said here to other manifestations of loss of control.

HOW DOES CRYING MANIFEST ITSELF AND WHAT DOES IT SIGNIFY?

Physiologically one finds an increase of lacrimation, there are facial changes, including some grimacing, dilated conjunctival veins, a reddened nose, and swollen eyelids. There is usually sobbing and, often, a loss of general tone and purposive movement. There may be wailing or whining, sometimes even screaming. Lacrimation without emotional changes is not considered to be weeping, nor are the motor manifestations without accompaniment of tears.

Although there are different interpretations of what crying signifies, most authors are agreed that it denotes a state of helplessness. In the infant and young child, unable to help himself, weeping thus becomes a plea for adult intervention. This is not necessarily always the case, however, in the older child or the adult. Although they, too, are overwhelmed by helplessness, they may perceive crying as a relief in itself; or they may be so embarrassed by the fact that they are crying that they may strive to hide their tears from others as well as the subjective state that brought forth these tears, which in turn may increase their burden.

WHO ARE THE CRYING PATIENTS?

Under what circumstances do adult patients in general hospitals cry? Usually one finds that men are more reluctant to resort to crying than women, but they too will cry on occasion. It may happen when the pain they must bear is simply more than they can endure. It may also happen if they have lost the existence or function of a body part which is of especial significance to them.

Women, in addition to the above circumstances which hold true for them as well, are found to cry when they want to draw attention to their pain or discomfort and when they are separated from their loved ones. They may cry because they are afraid of what will happen to them, both when they know and when they don't know what the future holds in store for them. They may also cry after having been told the good news that "It is all over", that "It's a boy" or that the results of the biopsy were negative.

Men and women of the older age group or those with progressive neurological or cerebral disorders may cry easily and sometimes for no apparent reason. The same is true of patients who are suffering from transient depressions, such as a woman after childbirth; it may be true of patients who are on the road to becoming seriously depressed.

THE NURSE'S RESPONSE

Sometimes a patient begins to cry in the course of discussing matters of concern to him with the nurse, which may give the nurse the feeling that he would not be crying were it not for her clumsiness.

How do nurses tend to respond to crying patients? Usually they focus on the crying itself rather than on the attending circumstances. Thus, they may explicitly *encourage* a patient to continue with his crying, because it is "good for him." Or they may ask him to *stop* crying for, after all, the patient is a grown man (or woman). Sometimes the nurse asks the patient *why* he is crying, anticipating, of course, that he has the answer to this question.

Why does the nurse seem to prefer addressing the patient directly with respect to his crying rather than evaluating first what the crying may signify in a particular case? One reason for this may be, as was discussed in the beginning of this paper, that nurses (and other people too) feel exceedingly uncomfortable in the presence of crying adults.

Somehow we feel that if a person, regardless whether he is of this or another culture, must resort to crying, something must be amiss; someone, most likely we ourselves, must have, unwittingly perhaps, let this person down in some unforgivable way. We tend to feel guilty, then, when we are confronted by a crying adult and we feel vaguely responsible for his misery. We also feel that we should be doing something about his obvious suffering; we should be able to take it away from him, but we don't quite know how. We feel especially helpless if we do not know what his crying is all about, or if his circumstances are such that, in our estimation, he has very good reason to cry. In the latter case we may also feel deep sympathy with the patient, but are at a loss as to how to express it, for fear it may make him feel even worse.

In some instances the crying we witness seems to denote self-pity or seems somehow to be incongruous with the existing situation. In this case we may feel an upsurge of irritation or impatience, two more emotions that we do not feel free to express openly.

We can see, then, that the nurse, when she deals directly with the patient's crying, is really responding to her own feeling of discomfort. And what does this do to the patient? Well, he may be embarrassed, for he may not wish anyone to know that he is upset. He may be annoyed, for he may not share the nurse's opinion that crying is something he should indulge in; on the other hand, he may want to be free to cry if and when he pleases. He may be bewildered, for how else was he to let the nurse know that he is in need of help? Or, if he is already somewhat shaken about the fact that he seems to be crying out of context, as it were, her pointing a finger at this may strengthen his belief that something serious is amiss with him.

WHAT CAN THE NURSE DO?

What else might the nurse do then? I think that she needs to assess first whether the crying denotes a message which the patient is trying to convey to her: a message such as "Look, I am in pain, do something about it," or "Look at the mess I am in; I am literally soaking in my drainage." If the message is clear enough so that she is reasonably sure of it, the nurse merely needs to convey to the patient that she has understood. Thus, she might state: "I see you are having quite a bit of pain; it is just about time for your next injection." Or "I can see why you are uncomfortable; I will be right back to change your dressings and freshen you up a bit."

What about the patient who attempts to hide his crying from the nurse and who is desperately trying to retain or at least regain his composure? I believe that it is the nurse's obligation to assist him in this effort to the best of her ability. Thus, she may aid him to stop the flow of tears by discretely moving his box of tissues closer within his reach. She may initiate a topic of conversation quite unrelated to his current concern. She may even, if this is not too taxing for his physical well-being, ask him to help her with a task she knows he can do well, such as the crossword puzzle of today's paper.

If a patient cries from the sheer effort he or she is making to cope with intense discomfort or pain, it is also better not to focus directly on the crying. Instead, the nurse might let the patient know that the painful procedure he is undergoing will soon be over (of course, only if this is actually the case). She might sustain him in his effort by remarks such as "You are doing very well—keep it up just a little while longer." She might try to divert him from his suffering by encouraging him to participate actively in the task at hand; thus, she might remind him to keep taking deep breaths or keep trying to relax. Whenever possible, the nurse should give him an opportunity to hold onto her hand. If this is not feasible she should try by some means to convey her "thereness" through physical contact, so that he may derive added strength from her.

If the nurse knows that the patient is crying because of a past or anticipated loss, she might indicate to him through verbal or nonverbal means that she is available in case he would like to talk to her about what troubles him. I realize that many nurses are reluctant to take this step for fear that the patient might take them up on their offer. For, suppose he opens up and unburdens himself to the nurse, what is she then to do with this burden, how can she take it away from him and relieve him of its pain? It may be helpful to the nurse if she reminds herself every so often that the patient's burden is his own and will remain his regardless of how skillful her intervention. All she is asked to do is to lend him support so that he can summon the necessary strength to take his burden upon himself as his own, so that he can bear it, and, hopefully, eventually assimilate it as part of his life.

Usually, as the patient begins to talk to the nurse about his past or impending loss, his crying will subside, but only for a while. In facing his loss and attempting to come to grips with it, he cannot help but collide with its full impact and with the many implications it will have for him in the future. It may well be, therefore, that the crying may resume, perhaps even more forcefully.

There is no need, however, for the nurse to feel guilty about this, as if she had made the patient feel worse or had failed to help him. True, he may be suffering more now than he did before he began to talk, but he is not suffering because of her. She has not forced him into talking about his loss, but had left it up to him whether he wanted to make use of her assistance.

Even though the patient's account of the loss and its meaning to him may well be interrupted by periods of crying, there is no need for the nurse to talk about the crying itself. Instead she can merely wait until it subsides sufficiently for the patient to continue where he has left off. If, because he is crying, she has difficulty understanding his words, she can ask him to repeat his statement or repeat it herself in order to make sure that she has heard him right.

Sometimes a patient, though not hiding the fact that he or she is crying, will give no clues to the nurse as to what the crying is all about. In this case the nurse will need to press the patient a little bit as to the circumstances that have elicited the crying. Without appearing too sympathetic or unsympathetic she might merely ask the patient to tell her what happened, and then try to get as full a description of the event that precipitated the crying including the patient's participation in the event. Only then should she try to find out more about the patient's thoughts and feelings. For, if she first went after the patient's thoughts and feelings concerning what to her is an unknown quantity, she would merely be pouring oil on the existing fire without being any closer to discovering its source.

It may well be, however, that the patient is unable or unwilling to follow through on the nurse's suggestion at this time. If, after a reasonable waiting period, the patient persists with his crying without indicating the reason for it, the nurse might let him know that she is still in the dark and that there is little she can do for him unless she has some idea as to what is upsetting him. She might suggest to him that he try to compose himself and that she will be back in a little while and then, perhaps, he can tell her what it is all about.

WHEN CRYING SEEMS TO BE WITHOUT CAUSE

What might be the most suitable approach to a patient who complains to the nurse that he is crying without wanting to do so, without knowing why he is crying, and at the most inopportune times? This is usually an indication that some aspects of the patient's unconscious are clamoring to be recognized by him. It may be a sign that the patient is depressed, but does not in itself indicate the degree of the depression. On the other hand, it may merely indicate a phase of letdown after a prolonged effort or waiting period which was followed by a joyful climax, such as childbirth or test results that indicated no malignancy.

The nurse, unless she has had specialized training in maternal and child care or psychiatric nursing, cannot expect of herself to be able to assess and weigh the seriousness of this seemingly inappropriate crying. It is therefore imperative that she report it to someone better qualified to make this judgment. Before she leaves the patient in order to do so, she can try to elicit from him more specific information as to the time of day when the crying occurs and also its duration, and whether it happens when the patient is alone or in the presence of specific people and if so, which ones. She can also let the patient know that his crying will be reported to his physician and that, in the meantime, the patient should not hesitate to call on the nurse whenever he feels the need of her presence.

WHEN CRYING HAS AN ORGANIC CAUSE

With patients whose emotions are labile due to organic changes in the brain and nervous system, no issue should be made of the crying, unless they themselves want to talk about it. It is hard to set general guidelines for these patients, for the exact meaning of the crying may be clear to the nurse only after she has come to know the patient pretty well.

It may be that he merely overreacts to a given situation and that with a few words he can gently be diverted into thinking about other, more pleasant matters. It may be that he is tired from the effect of too many stimuli on his system. In this case, it may be best to take him to his bed and encourage him to rest for a little while. It also may be that he feels rather sorry for himself, for he sees little improvement, if any, in spite of conscientious efforts on his part to exercise his inert and unresponsive limbs. I think that in this case the nurse needs to acknowledge to the patient that his is not an easy lot and that it is hard to persevere in the light of no tangible signs of improvement. At the same time she will have to encourage him to keep up the good work, however, because whether it shows or not it does have positive effects which he would sorely miss if he were to stop his efforts.

It may also be that the patient as yet has not had enough opportunity to talk about his condition, about the ways in which it has changed his life, and about the fact that this suffering has opened up many previous and improperly healed painful memories. If so, the nurse might arrange to see him for short periods daily or at least several times a week, in which he can feel free to talk to her about his present state or his past sufferings. It does not matter on which he dwells longer. Unless he has dealt to his satisfaction with the unfinished business of his past, he will not be able to assimilate his current state. On the other hand, his current state may put past events into new perspective for him which will enable him finally to come to grips with them.

Why does Dr. Ujhely repeatedly say not to focus your attention on the crying? Does this mean to always pretend that the crying is not happening?

What options does she give the nurse to choose from when confronted with a crying patient? Can you state three? If not, glance back through the article. How might the nurse's feelings influence which option of nursing action is taken?

Refer to page 57 for your original answers to questions and see if there has been any change in your responses.

11.

Helping the Person Adjust to Stress

Jo Anna A. Green

Recall some newly admitted patients that you have seen. What behavior did they show that you suspect was caused by anxiety?

If you have ever been a patient in the hospital try to recall how you felt. Did you miss such creature comforts as a cup of coffee whenever you wished, an aspirin easily available in a cupboard, a newspaper delivery, or maybe just being able to adjust the temperature of your room without having to consult strangers? Read about some more changes.

What is meant by "preventive medicine"? Does this term pertain only to techniques that help prevent physical disease or can it also be used as a name for those techniques that help individuals to deal with the stresses of daily living?

The nurse who cares for hospitalized people is, I believe, practicing preventive medicine in the latter sense. For she is helping these people maintain their emotional balance—their mental health—in a stress-filled situation.

Each year thousands of people are admitted to general medical/surgical hospitals. Is not each of these persons involved in a personal crisis? Is it not wise and humane as well as professional for the nurse to provide the assistance each person needs to help him through one of the most stressful situations of his life?

Sigmund Freud is known as the Father of Psychiatry. But Hans Selye defined the stress syndrome in terms that made the modern world aware of what constitutes stress, how many times it occurs in each 24 hours, and what transpires physiologically each time it occurs. The nurse who understands what produces stress can do much to alleviate it for the hospitalized person and, perhaps, shorten the time it takes for the person to recover.

When a person is admitted to the hospital he is virtually stripped of all independence. If he's acutely ill, he may be relieved to have decisions made for him. But suppose he is suffering from only slight discomfort: What then should be his reaction?

The label "patient" carries a role with it. The person so labeled is expected to act like every other patient. Thus is the nurse relieved of the effort of treating the patient as a person who has unique anxieties, needs, and goals.

There is entirely too much talk about the patient "adjusting" to the hospital, and what a problem he is to the nursing staff if he does not "adjust." Is it desirable for him to turn over nearly all his responsibilities for self-care and decision-making to others? *Should* he become so well "adjusted" that he comes to see the hospital routine as normal and the outside world as abnormal?

The answer is obvious: We should not expect this of persons who are hospitalized. Our role is to help them not to become "patients" but to maintain an optimum level of mental health as well as physical health, and to return as quickly as possible to the tasks of daily living. To do this we must be able to recognize and to ease the many stresses that hospitalization imposes.

These stresses start with admission. In most hospitals the admission procedure produces all kinds of negative feelings, including excessive anxiety. At a time when the person is worried about his physical well-being, he is expected to sit quietly in the admitting office and provide reams and reams of data: his birth date, his parents' birth dates, his place of birth, their places of birth, his marital status, etc., etc. He is bombarded by questions, many of which are asked in an authoritarian way, and seem threatening. Later in the admission procedure, he must disrobe, put on a revealing hospital gown, undergo laboratory tests, and submit to a physical examination. Finally he finds himself in a room with a perfect stranger with whom he must live 24 hours a day, and the two of them are "expected" to get along together.

Certainly some means can be found to ease these procedures! Perhaps portions of the data required on admission could be obtained from the individual later, when he is less anxiety-ridden. Perhaps arrangements could be made so that the nurse who will be in charge of this person's care could meet him at once, spend some time with him, get to know him, and thereby gain some understanding of how to help him.

The nurse who desires that her care be truly therapeutic *listens* to what the hospitalized person tells her through his words, attitude, and actions. She lets *him* determine the kinds of questions he wants answered, and the pace at which he wants them answered. She does not, for instance, "do a beautiful piece of teaching" about a test or procedure in a situation in which this isn't desirable.

It is also important that the nurse convey clearly to the hospitalized person the idea that she has time to listen to him. If she always seems rushed, if she never goes into his room unless she has something in her hands or there is a physical procedure to be done, she certainly doesn't encourage the patient to talk. Oftentimes, listening is much more stressful than "doing things." This may be the real reason why so many nurses today claim that they are too busy to "spend time listening."

Another means by which the nurse can reduce anxiety is to tell the hospitalized person how much time she plans to spend with him (for a particular procedure), and when she will return to his room. This is especially important with the person who has been using his call light almost continuously. The nurse can anticipate some of his needs by careful observation. Is his liquid handy? Is the bed adjusted comfortably? Would he like to use the urinal or bedpan while she is there?

Surely the nurse can't help but realize that hospitalization has elements of stress in it for every person, and that this stress affects the *whole* person—mind and emotions as well as body. The nurse who understands this has taken the first step toward carrying out a truly therapeutic role in the lives of those persons who are under her care in the hospital.

What specific actions were suggested in order to help patients maintain an optimum level of mental health as well as physical health? List four specific actions the nurse can take and indicate which ones you have carried out for a patient during the past month.

Now think about how you might prepare a patient for admission to the hospital. Do you believe that forewarned is forearmed? You have learned how to prepare patients for surgery and to be concerned with their anxiety. How can nurses take an active part in preparing patients for their hospital experience and resultant anxiety?

As nurses are becoming more involved with prevention in the home as well as in physician's offices this becomes a pertinent question. Will some of the same guidelines that we use in preparing patients for surgery apply to preparing patients for hospitalization? See the articles in Part IV. Children are being routinely prepared in some doctor's offices but adults are usually just told the time and place to arrive. How could you change this situation?

12.
Developing the Difficult Patient

Donald I. Peterson

The following article is an autobiography and shows you an evaluation regarding the physical and emotional care given during long-term hospitalization. Studying the article now may help you prevent such difficulties for future patients.

Everyone who has responsibility for the care of patients should know the most effective ways to develop the "difficult patient." Several well established principles and simple techniques, if conscientiously applied, will nearly always insure success.

A difficult patient often is described as demanding, uncooperative, unresponsive to treatment, unappreciative, or generally unlikable.

Actually, a difficult patient is one whose needs are not met—emotional or physical or both. With the current emphasis upon emotional support, the unmet needs are more likely to be phsycial than emotional, especially when the patient is totally incapcitated.

The purpose of the difficult patient, of course, is to meet a need which exists in any well organized hospital. Every nursing unit should have at least one for how can the "good" be identified if there is no "bad" patient for comparison? Without those who excel in "difficultness," some everyday, run-of-the-mill, nongood, nonbad patients might be incorrectly classified as difficult—especially if they required lots of nursing care.

Sometimes the difficult patient's unique contribution is to those members of the health team who are frustrated and anxious. This common but often unrecognized need—for someone to whom they can feel superior—is mentioned by Barker, Wright, and others. William Gellman reports that a frustrated person can maintain his self-esteem by regarding disabled persons as if they were inferior.

The difficult patient, then, assuming a role that is hard to fill in any other way, is of inestimable value to the neurotic nurse, the anxious attendant, and the frustrated physician.

With the necessity for difficult patients clearly established, one must learn the most efficient method to produce an adequate supply of them.

SUBJECT CHARACTERISTICS

The first consideration is proper subject selection. Not everyone can be made into a difficult patient and, even among those who can, difficultness is induced much more readily in some subjects than in others.

Total or near total incapacity is desirable because the greater a patient's dependence and nursing needs, the easier it is to implement the program. Besides, the entirely incapacitated patient will cooperate with the program because he can do so little to counteract it.

A long-term, serious illness is best—one that does not progress rapidly in either direction. The acutely ill patient usually is a poor subject for he cannot be relied upon to be consistently difficult since his condition changes rapidly.

An existing depression is helpful but not essential because depression usually can be stimulated readily by the same measures that produce difficultness.

Authoritative, successful persons frequently respond well, because it is particularly hard for them to accept complete dependence on others.

PERSONNEL CHARACTERISTICS

The next step, selection of nursing and ancillary personnel, is almost as important as patient choice.

Unconcern about meeting patient needs should characterize those persons who care for him most of the time.

General maladjustment to life qualifies one to develop a patient's difficultness, and, in turn, to experience relief of one's own frustration by so doing. Although many hospital employees have been taught not to "identify" with the patient, they unknowingly may identify their own emotions of frustration and ineffectiveness with the helplessness of the patient and hate him for it. This aversion identification facilitates the program.

Dissatisfaction with the profession.

Length of experience. Other things being equal, then, a senior student or a graduate nurse seems more qualified than a younger nurse to develop difficultness.

TEAM APPROACH

After patient and key personnel have been chosen, the program can be started immediately, but it must be well organized around the team approach for greatest success.

The regular nursing conferences offer the most auspicious means to orient personnel. Employ psychiatric terms to place the approach to the patient in a scientific framework; someone may be motivated to write a paper about the patient's abnormal psychology. Visual aids can reinforce your teaching. Showing the excellent film "Mrs. Difficult Needs a Nurse" should convince staff members that the needs of a completely immobilized patient are emotional rather than physical.

Make it very clear that the patient is afraid he will die and that all he needs, therefore, is to know that someone is near. Point out that the patient does not really want what he asks for; he only wants verbal reassurance. If he makes a statement, he does not mean what he *says* but something entirely different, something which only a Sigmund Freud ever could possibly decipher and interpret.

Never underestimate the contribution which the patient's physician can make. A question from the nurse—"Can't you do something about the man in Room 107?"—will put the physician on the defensive. He may reply, "We'll do a porcelain test. He's an old crock anyway."

This dialogue not only verifies that the patient is less ill than he thinks he is, but helps maintain team morale—everyone is working together toward the same objective with the doctor leading the team.

If he is a surgeon, he may become discouraged if the patient does not respond to surgery, and may visit him less and less often. While desertion of the patient by his doctor is certainly helpful, usually one cannot depend upon this assistance for long because he may refer the patient to someone interested in rehabilitation of the chronically ill. And *this* can threaten the entire development of a difficult patient.

Difficultness should come along nicely if everyone is closely supervised and if one adds those extra refinements which can be introduced in any therapeutic community. Hospital routine already is geared to depersonalize the patient. Having a numbered identification band applied to the wrist and being designated by room number rather than by name initiates this process. Now, give the patient a shrunken, coarse-textured gown that gaps open in the back. Having no clothes below the waist undermines dignity and self-confidence unless the patient happens to be a nudist. While such depersonalization can pave the way for more complete depersonalization, it is not sufficient in itself to develop difficultness. Further measures such as objectivity, are required. Always speak *about* a patient, never *to* him.

For instance, say to the orderly, "I don't believe he will get too cold if you open the window."

The orderly might properly answer, "No, I don't think he will. It seems warm to me." The orderly might then ask, "Don't you think he needs a shave today? He looks a bit bushy."

Another very effective approach: "I think you should give him the bedpan. It's about the time of day he usually goes."

Make the patient realize that he can make *no* decisions regarding his care because this might upset the orderly progress of scheduled routine.

Remember, too, that this patient has family and friends interested in his condition. Why not share encouraging developments by saying to his visitors, "He is so much better today. He had an enema yesterday, with excellent results."

Never ask the patient how he feels; tell him. Assume that he does not know how he should feel since he probably has never been hospitalized before.

Do not accept the patient as a person. If he is completely helpless, possibly he already doubts the reality of his "body image," has little feeling of security, almost no feeling of accomplishment, and not very much to look forward to. If you remove his feeling of acceptance, any vestige of confidence he has in himself will be gone.

To polish the luster of this now quite difficult patient, reinforce his growing feeling of worthlessness by mentioning a patient in the next room who has been unconscious for six months—such a "good" patient who never says a word; express your concern that your patient is unable even to feed himself. Should he ask to be moved because his weight-bearing areas are painfully tender from long-continued pressure against a wet, wrinkled sheet, remind him of your own fatigue and of how you wish *you* could lie down to rest and not move a muscle.

Pain erodes morale rather effectively so let your patient who is in an uncomfortable position wait a long time before you move him. You might wonder aloud whether he actually is in pain. Your last paralyzed patient, who was no trouble at all, could not feel a thing. Encourage him to be forbearing. After all, you *do* have other patients to take care of.

When his pain is severe enough to make him cry for relief, he can be classified as "demanding"; the program is nearly complete.

Humor is a useful adjunct provided you smile or even laugh at just the right time. Talk and laugh with others in subdued tones that can be heard but not understood by the patient. It makes little difference what you are laughing about. If you do it somewhat furtively, the patient will think you are laughing at him—especially if he needs a shave and a haircut and is on the bedpan.

Finally, point out his guilt. Suggest that if he had lived right, been honest, and had morals at least the equivalent of an alley cat's, he might not be in this terrible condition. Has he ever wondered why this misfortune came to *him*? Has he considered that there must be a reason for his suffering?

At this juncture you should be able to call this patient "difficult." If not, check his vital signs to see if he is still responding.

These techniques can produce difficult patients. I know. I've been one.

React to the statement in the beginning of Dr. Peterson's article "With the current emphasis upon emotional support, the unmet needs are more likely to be physical than emotional . . . ." Then consider how you react to criticism in general and why.

This article is criticizing nursing care in the same way that difficult, demanding patients do with their behavior. He is saying "You have failed to make me happy. You are doing something wrong." How can we learn to use this criticism constructively instead of defensively? How can we deal with our feelings of failure that Dr. Peterson says causes us to depersonalize our care and avoid the patient?

13.

A Patient's Concern with Death

Joan M. Baker
Karen C. Sorensen

The following article was placed in this section of the book because the focus is mainly on communication skills in a difficult situation. Since 1963 when this article was published, much work has been done in the area of death and grief. Part III of this book deals with this subject in depth. After reading Part III, you might wish to return to this article and identify the stages of grief that the first nurse – Ann Smith – and the patient, Mr. J each are in.

If you have begun examining your feelings regarding death and your own prejudices about how you think people should react and behave, this article will help you try out your thoughts and feelings.

On your busy morning rounds, you stop by Mr. Jones' bed. He reaches for your hand and, as he takes it, says, "Nurse, I know I'm dying. Will it be today?"

Mr. Jones has been critically ill and appears exhausted. He looks directly at you, and the silence that follows his question suddenly becomes painful. Should you discuss this with him or remain silent? How can you help Mr. Jones? What could you say? Many questions flash across your mind as the silence continues and Mr. Jones awaits your answer.

In whatever way you decide to respond to Mr. Jones, there are several factors which will influence your decision. One is why you think Mr. Jones asked you this question. In other words, what is your perception of Mr. Jones' behavior? Do you believe he expects you to have an answer? Perhaps you feel that this is his way of letting you know he is afraid and wants to talk about his fear. Maybe you think he is testing you to find out if you will answer the same as others. Just what does he expect of you?

Other factors which will influence your response to Mr. Jones will be some of your own past experiences related to death and what dying means to you. Maybe talking about death makes you feel sad and inadequate because you have not been able to face and explore your own past experiences related to death. Perhaps to you, death is a personal experience which you feel should not be discussed with others or which should only be discussed with clergymen or doctors. What do you think happens to people when they die?

The nurse realizes that some of her patients may not yet have assigned their own meaning to death, although death may be near. It is important therefore that the discussion should be patient-centered and without the nurse's trying to interject her philosophy into the structure the patient is building. If free discussion is to be maintained, the nurse must not censor ideas which the patient may be presenting.

Many nurses have never pondered and formulated their own ideas about death before being confronted with a question similar to the one asked by Mr. Jones. This indeed is unfortunate and causes many nurses to direct their energies toward helping themselves in the situation rather than the patient.

A person is likely to feel more at ease when he is allowed to explore the meaning that death has for him and to arrive eventually at his own philosophy.

We have pointed out how the nurse's perception of the patient's behavior, combined with her own past experiences and philosophy concerning death, can affect her response to a patient. These factors will determine how the nurse feels when the patient brings up the subject of death. Each nurse will experience a variety of feelings. One nurse's predominant feeling may be confidence in her ability to help the patient communicate effectively about his thoughts and feelings. Another nurse may feel very threatened when the patient brings up such an emotionally charged subject. Thus, she may interfere with the patient's communication while attempting to make herself feel more comfortable.

When a nurse cannot comfortably discuss the subject of death with a patient, she may attempt to terminate the discussion in various ways. Mr. Jones has just asked the nurse if she thinks he will die that day. The nurse might respond by:

• Moralizing to the patient: "You shouldn't talk that way, Mr. Jones. No one knows when he will die." In effect, this nurse is telling Mr. Jones that it is wrong for him to talk about his death.

• Stating facts or possible facts which disagree with the feelings the patient is expressing: "I don't think you're going to die today, Mr. Jones. Let me take your pulse. Yes, it's strong and steady and your color is good. This isn't the end of you." This nurse is disregarding the feelings of the patient and using physiological facts to prove to the patient that his concern is not necessary.

• Denying directly the fact that the patient may die: "No, I don't think you'll die today or even tomorrow." This nurse's response discourages further communication by terminating the discussion with her own opinion.

• Philosophizing to the patient: "No one really knows what the future holds for him. It is up to each of us to have faith. There will be a tomorrow." Here the nurse states her own philosophy about life and death before giving the patient a chance to formulate his own.

• Changing the subject: "Who's that in the picture on your night stand?" This nurse avoids answering the patient and at the same time is showing disrespect for the patient's feelings by ignoring the question.

• Referring the patient to another person: "I am unable to tell you that. The doctor is better able to tell you what your condition is." Here the nurse is telling the patient that nurses aren't as able to talk with the patient as doctors are.

• Kidding the patient out of expressing further feelings: "Oh, come on now. You're going to outlive me." This nurse is making light of a very serious matter.

• Avoiding the question by silence or turning away from the patient. By her silence, the nurse indicates she cannot or will not discuss the matter, and she may busy herself in some activity such as cleaning out a nightstand drawer. (This silence is different from the one in which the nurse is looking at the patient understandingly and encouraging him to go on in the conversation.)

These examples show how a nurse can terminate a conversation and manipulate the patient into a position where his expression of feelings becomes secondary to her own comfort. In many of the examples, the nurse is verbalizing her own ideas instead of exploring those of the patient. In others, she may be prompting the patient to feel guilty about his attempt to talk about death. In all these situations the nurse is saying, "Stop talking about dying." While she may want to help the patient, the nurse's inability to tolerate further discussion may indicate to the patient that she is not interested in him. Such responses force the patient to face this problem alone or to keep seeking for someone who will help him think through his feelings.

How might a nurse participate more effectively with a patient in discussing death? The following situation illustrates some basic principles related to helping the patient communicate his feelings.

Ann Smith is a nurse on the ward where Mr. Jones is a patient. She enters his room and the following interaction takes place:

Mr. J (weakly): "Oh, hello, Miss Smith." The patient's tone of voice offers the nurse a clue.

Miss S: "Hello, Mr. Jones. I thought I'd drop in for a while and see how you are feeling." The nurse pauses and allows the patient to respond.

Mr. J: "Well, this will probably be your last chance." The patient drops another vague clue.

Miss S: "I don't quite understand what you mean." Instead of jumping to conclusions about what the patient might mean, Miss Smith asks for clarification—she is inviting the patient to speak directly about his concern.

Mr. J: "I'm sinking fast. Do you think I'll die today?" Mr. Jones now speaks directly about his problem and asks the nurse for a direct answer to it.

Miss S: "Why do you ask that, Mr. Jones?" Miss Smith avoids a direct answer to the question and instead invites the patient to express himself further. The nurse stays with the subject rather than terminating it as in the previous examples. The nurse could have been more direct in answering the patient by preceding her comment by, "I don't know, Mr. Jones."

Mr. J: "I'm so weak, I can barely take a drink of water by myself." The patient is just beginning to discuss some of the reasons related to his concern about dying. He waits to see what the nurse will do now.

Miss S: "Yes?" She encourages him to continue—her tone tells him that she is ready to continue listening to him.

Mr. J: "I was pretty sick for a long time. The doctor told my wife that death knocked at my door." Mr. Jones is telling Miss Smith that the doctor implied that death was close at hand.

Miss S: "Yes, I remember." The nurse indicates she is still listening and refrains from making an interpretation.

Mr. J: "I'm glad I didn't go then, but I'm afraid I will now, even though I'm supposed to be better." Mr. Jones is glad to be alive but wonders if he is out of danger.

Miss S: "You're afraid you're going to die now?" Miss Smith, quite sure by now that her patient feels more capable of pursuing the subject, restates in more direct terms what Mr. Jones has said—asking for further elaboration about his feelings.

Mr. J: "Yes, I haven't slept for two nights, I've been so afraid." Patient relates what this fear is doing to hamper his recovery. His statement begins to point out to the nurse some action which will be helpful.

Miss S: "You haven't even been able to sleep?" Again, the nurse reflects on the patient's comment.

Mr. J: "No I'm afraid I'm going to die. You know, Mother used to say that we each have an angel and when we die this angel goes with us." Mr. Jones again restates his fear and tells the nurse of an idea he has heard about dying.

Miss S: "Oh?" The nurse refrains from commenting directly on this idea.

Mr. J: "Do you think she was right?" (Looks intently at Miss Smith.) The patient is now asking the nurse to be more direct and to communicate her ideas to him.

Miss S (ponderingly): "Well, I don't know, Mr. Jones. What do you think about it?" While Miss Smith responds directly, she remains noncommittal and helps Mr. Jones to explore his ideas further. (Miss Smith realized that what she thought about Mr. Jones' idea was not important, but what was important, was to continue to express interest in the idea and allow the patient to explore his feelings.)

Mr. J: "I think maybe she was but I'm so tired. I can hardly talk or think about it." Mr. Jones indicates that he, too, believes in the idea he presented as his mother's. He feels too tired to talk further.

Miss S: "Would you feel safer in going to sleep if I stayed with you for a while?" Miss Smith, taking advantage of the information the patient has given her, suggests a therapeutic nursing action.

Mr. J: "You mean sit right by my bed?" He asks for further clarification and indicates a need for closeness.

Miss S: "Yes." Miss Smith recognizes this need and together they have planned the nursing action.

Mr. J: "I think I'll try it." (He turns on his side.) "I don't feel so afraid when someone is with me." Mr. Jones accepts the nursing action and indicates his fear has subsided somewhat.

Three principles have been formulated from the previous interaction. It is hoped, they may lead to helpful therapeutic action in situations where a patient shows concern about death. These principles are not only applicable to discussing death, but may also be used in situations where the patient is attempting to investigate other emotionally charged areas.

- Don't close the door with your own doubts or fears.

When the patient expresses an idea or opinion and the nurse explores this by asking him for clarification, by asking for more iformation, and by reflecting back the patient's idea or opinion, and does not state her own, then the patient is allowed a greater degree of freedom in expressing himself and has more opportunity to explore, clarify, and define his own thinking.

However, when the nurse states her own views about what the patient has expressed, which either support or oppose the idea or opinion of the patient, then there will be less opportunity for the patient to explore freely, clarify, and define his own thinking.

- Lead the patient but don't drag him.

When a patient is vague in his communication, the nurse can help him communicate more clearly and directly by asking the patient what he means, summarizing what she thinks the patient means and asking the patient to validate her summary, or by indicating her own lack of understanding of the patient's communication.

However, when the nurse responds as if she knew what the patient was attempting to communicate, communication may remain vague, distorted, and incomplete.

• Find a mutual goal.

When the nurse and patient pursue the same goal, or attempt to solve the same problem, it is more likely that the goal will be attained or the problem solved to their mutual satisfaction.

However, when the nurse and patient are pursuing separate goals or problems, blocking and conflict may often be the outcome with resulting mutual dissatisfaction.

The Reverend Peter S. Raible of the University Unitarian Church in Seattle said in a sermon on the theology of death, "In an age when death is so assiduously avoided it is perhaps natural that many are allowed to end their lives in ignorance of what is happening to them or, even more likely, in a sham pretense carried on by relative, patient, and physician alike that death is not at hand."

Nurses, too, are guilty of these offenses. Death is but one phase of life; it is the experience which all of us are destined for from birth. Nurses are becoming increasingly skilled in helping people discuss and meet all phases of life's progression—birth, childhood, adolescence, adulthood, aging. Death—the next phase in the natural progression of life—is too often avoided as a topic of discussion.

We deal physically with the dying and the dead, but do not give the living the natural opportunity to discuss this experience adequately. We need to become more alert to what the patient is saying. Patients may bring up the subject of death in various ways. Let them have the opportunity to express themselves without censure.

Often nurses express concern about harming patients if they discuss death with them. Nurses also express insecurity about exploring this area because they may be asked unanswerable questions. We need to recognize when patients are indicating a desire to explore and also to realize that we cannot give omniscient answers to questions concerning death. Instead, nurses can help each patient formulate his own philosophy of death by keeping their responses free from personal prejudices. We must always keep in mind that some persons may not wish to discuss the subject of death even when its presence is imminent. That is each person's prerogative.

The difficult part of death is not the act of dying itself, we believe but in preparing for coming death. There are no magic words or pat routines by which one person can help another to adjust to dying. Rather each occasion calls for a personal assessment and decision by the person in the position to help.

Role play the dialogue in the article in order to get a feel for
Mr. J's mood. Do not hurry Miss S's responses but allow her to
pause and ponder before speaking. Then for practice, you might
act out the conversation between Mr. J and Miss S using Mr. J's
comments and responding spontaneously as Miss S. Find out
how you would respond and why.

For practice, you might act out the conversation between Mr. J
and Miss S using Mr. J's comments and responding spontaneously
as Miss S. Find out how you would respond and why.

14.

Reflections on ''Intensive'' Care

Helen J. Hammes

*The following four patients will present you with real life
situations. Can you try to help them with their emotional
needs? After each patient is described, stop and write down
exactly what you would say and do for the patient if you
were his nurse.*

Mrs. Larson, a 43-year-old housewife, was in the second post operative day
following a mitral valve replacement; nine-year-old Chucky was in his third day
following a second stage Blalock-Hanlon procedure; Mr. Gregory, a young
farmer, had just come from the recovery room after having an amputation of his
entire right arm and shoulder following a farm accident; and Mrs. White, another
middle-aged housewife, was in her second day following replacement of an aortic
valve. They were typical patients in the intensive care unit where I worked for
the summer.

In essence, the nursing care assignment for each of these patients read:
Observe and record vital signs every half hour; check venous pressure hourly;
observe and record urine volume, specific gravity, and pH every two hours;
intermittent positive pressure breathing and blow bottles every two hours; help
patient turn, cough, and hyperventilate every two hours, with tracheal
suctioning as needed; replace chest drainage with blood; maintain intravenous
drip at a specified hourly rate; replace gastric drainage with replacement fluid;
administer drugs.

It was a busy place. Surgeons were in and out, checking on patients, conferring with the nurses, and occasionally adding to or changing orders. Everyone focused on solving these patients' crucial physical problems. The care was expert, the concern real. But, in an intensive care unit, is that enough?

THE EMERGENCY TRACHEOSTOMY

Mrs. Larsen's breathing had become labored, despite frequent suctioning. Her nurse promptly called the surgeon, who examined Mrs. Larson and decided a tracheostomy was indicated. "The doctor is going to do a tracheostomy—cut a little hole in your neck—so you can breathe easier," the nurse hurriedly explained.

Because she was engrossed in preparing the tracheostomy equipment, the nurse seemed unaware of Mrs. Larson's frightened reaction to this perfunctory explanation. Although highly perceptive in noting physical signs, the nurse missed the anxious expression on her patient's face. She did not see Mrs. Larson's thin white hands clutch the sheet as if for support.

After Mrs. Larson's tracheostomy was performed, her husband came in to see her. Mr. Larson was unprepared for the sight of his wife with "a hole cut in her neck." He assumed this meant that his wife's critical condition was deteriorating. His concern and fear were reflected in his face and, unfortunately, Mrs. Larson saw it. Her own increasing fear was reinforced.

THE CARDIAC CHILD

Busy nurses, efficient in attending to Chucky's physical needs, found it almost necessary to withdraw emotionally from this demanding child. After spending considerable time and effort helping Chucky cough and turn, checking his chest drainage, and so on, it was frustrating to hear him cry out only seconds later, "Nurse, nurse, I want to be turned."

Under the best of circumstances Chucky was not an agreeable child. He had been overprotected and overcontrolled, and was emotionally immature for his age. Chucky had had six previous hospitalizations which had entailed not only major surgery, but lengthy and painful separation from his family as well. His demands could have been an attempt to control his anxiety. Taking time to consider some of these reasons behind Chucky's behavior would have made it easier to accept him and to help him acquire the feeling of control he seemed to need.

In the intense environment within the ICU, where relationships can be quickly damaged or cemented, quick insight is needed into the reasons behind one's own behavior as well as the patient's. His mother's visits were a real source of comfort to Chucky. But, according to hospital regulations, she was allowed to be with him only 10 minutes every hour until 8:00 P.M. One evening when

Chucky seemed especially fretful and demanding, the nurse caring for him wisely relaxed the rigid regulations. At 9:00 P.M. the float nurse who came in to relieve the regular nurse seemed disturbed to see that Chucky's mother was still there. "You shouldn't be here; visiting hours are over. You'll have to leave," she announced.

Understandably, Chucky and his mother were upset. As it happened, the float nurse had just finished assisting the cardiac arrest team and, despite their skilled efforts, it appeared unlikely that the patient would survive. It had been a traumatic experience for everyone.

Because she had participated in a situation where circumstances had been beyond medical control and failure seemed inevitable, the float nurse naturally enough experienced feelings of frustration and inadequacy. This may have accounted for her sharp rebuke to Chucky's mother and her seeming insensitivity to their feelings. Although the nurse's reactions were understandable, in this case they intruded and probably added to the anxiety which Chucky and his mother already felt.

THE AMPUTATION

A close watch had to be kept on Mr. Gregory's blood loss. His nurse gently changed the outer dressings on his massive wound, meticulously weighing them so she could replace his blood losses. She carefully observed his physical signs and symptoms, and showed intelligent concern for his excessive thirst. In all ways, she gave Mr. Gregory excellent physical care.

However, when Mr. Gregory attempted to communicate his anguish over the loss of his shoulder and arm, this same nurse became extremely uncomfortable, and hurriedly changed the subject. Another opportunity for Mr. Gregory, a normally reticent person, to express his overwhelming feelings came about quite by accident. While making rounds the head nurse remarked to Mr. Gregory's nurse, "They want to send us another patient, but we don't have one empty bed."

Mr. Gregory, hearing this, looked down at his mutilated body and whispered, "They can have my bed. I want to go."

At first the nurse did not comprehend the real meaning of his words, and she answered, "Everyone feels that way about the intensive care unit, Mr. Gregory. They all want to go." A moment later she realized his true meaning and protested awkwardly, "Oh, you mustn't speak like that. You're going to get well."

Mr. Gregory shook his head in despair and turned his face away.

THE COMPLAINER

Mrs. White was a very anxious patient. Although her vital signs indicated that she was progressing satisfactorily, she complained about physical symptoms almost constantly.

While the nurse was checking her apical pulse, Mrs. White might inquire, "Why is my heart beating so fast? Just listen to it pound! I didn't think it would do that after a new valve. I can even feel it pounding in my throat."

The nurse would explain to Mrs. White that her heart rate was within normal limits, the rhythm was regular, and the quality good. But Mrs. White never paid any attention, and a minute later would complain, "I feel as if I'm burning up. Feel my forehead. I must have a high fever. You'd better check my temperature." Again the nurse would truthfully but futilely answer, "Your temperature has come down nicely, Mrs. White."

Eventually, the nurses became impatient with Mrs. White's apparent inability to understand rational explanations, and answered her complaints with easy clichés: "You have nothing to worry about, Mrs. White. The doctors say you're doing very well. Try not to worry." Yet these same nurses would never have repeatedly employed ineffective nursing methods in attempting to meet Mrs. White's physical needs.

I do not intend in any way to devalue the importance of excellent physical care for patients in intensive care units, nor to imply that attention to patients' feelings is always overlooked. I intend only to point out the importance of attention to these patients' emotional needs with the same consistency, dedication, and skill used in meeting their physical needs. Of course, many nurses do acquire this ability and learn to give both physical and emotional care. Those who do give nursing care that is truly intensive.

What signs of anxiety did the nurse fail to observe in her patients?

Picture your hospital's Intensive Care Unit and list factors that contribute to sensory deprivation for the patients, such as lack of windows.

What could be done to remedy some of these problems?

Which, if any, of these same problems are present elsewhere in your hospital?

How do people react when deprived of their normal sensory stimulation?

Compare your solutions with others. These are good examples to bring to a group discussion for role playing. How would you handle the impatience felt by the nurse who is constantly being called by Chucky? How could you help Mr. Gregory grieve for the loss of his arm? For more information on grieving see the articles in Part III.

PART II

KNOWING YOUR AGES

Nurses need to concern themselves with the ages of their patients. A five year old, a 12 year old, a newborn, an elderly adult, and a pregnant woman all have different abilities and needs because of their ages. It is not possible to intuitively know these differences about age groups. Each of us is more familiar with some ages than others depending on our own age, life experiences, and ages of those close to us.

Perhaps there should be a new style of aging in the world today. Could it be that one of the reasons for the generation gap today is that grandparents have copped out? Young people are being deprived of knowing why their parents behave so peculiarly and why their grandparents say the things they do. In days past, grandparents taught the young about what the end of life was going to be. You looked at your mother, if you were a girl, and learned what it was like to be a bride and a young mother. Then you looked at your grandmother and you knew what it was like to be old. Children learned what it was to age and die while they were very small. They were prepared for the end of life at the beginning.

Today, grandparents, and old people in general, have something quite different to contribute. Their generation has seen the most change in the world and the young today need to learn that there has been change. Young people in this country are accused of not caring for their parents the way they would have in the old country. But old people in this country have been influenced by an American ideal of independence and autonomy . To many it seems that the most important thing in the world is to be independent. An aged person may live alone on the verge of starvation, but he is independent. Everyone who is aging has a chance to develop a new life style. Everyone who is working with old people can contribute to this new style of aging.

But even while being independent older people must think in terms of what they can do for other generations. If the style of aging is to be changed, then older people will have to take the lead by finding new ways to relate either to their own grandchildren or to someone else's. As long as youth feels no respect for age and young people in this country have no interest in old people (in seeing them or listening to them), there will be an enormous number of things in our society that are not being done but that could be done by old people.

Think of this as you read these articles related to growth and development and developmental tasks so that nursing care can be adapted to each individual's age.

THE YOUNG

15.

The Newborn: Transition to Extra-Uterine Life

*Helen W. Arnold, Nancy J. Putnam, Betty Lou Barnard,
Murdina M. Desmond, Arnold J. Rudolph*

*What does it mean to be "in limbo?" At best, this is a disquieting
feeling and not one we like to encourage. The helpless newborn
needs help through the transition state immediately after birth
more than at any other time. He is extremely vulnerable and
needs intensive nursing care. Human beings find that transition
periods occur throughout life. Help the newborn make a successful
transition and recognize that, as the newborn needs help, so do
others – in different ways – through the periods "in limbo".*

Transition is the period which bridges intra-uterine to extra-uterine life, a period through which every infant must pass if he is to survive and grow and develop normally. The newly born infant, like the astronaut, must make rapid physiologic changes to adjust to a new environment. The quiescent fetus in the uterus must pass through a series of six overlapping steps before he becomes fully adapted, ready for living in the air-breathing world.

Step one occurs with labor as the fetus receives stimulation from the changes in pressure brought to bear on his body by the contracting uterus and the loss of uterine volume with the rupture of the membranes. During the second step, the infant on delivery encounters an avalanche of new stimuli (gravity, light, sound, cold). In step three, the infant initiates air breathing. This is followed, in steps four and five, by profound changes in the function of organ systems and the reorganization of metabolic processes. The changes in function of organ systems consist of the initiation of respiration, the change from fetal to neonatal circulation, alterations of the hepatic and renal functions, and the passage of meconium. The sixth step, the reorganization of metabolic processes to achieve a level or steady state, includes induction of enzymes, changes in blood oxygen saturation, a diminution of postnatal acidosis, and recovery of neural tissues following the intense stimuli of labor and delivery. It is only after these changes in function and reorganization have taken place that the neonate can be said to be adapted to independent existence.

We became convinced that a transitional care nursery was necessary after making the surprising discovery that we knew little about the physical signs accompanying the transitional process, even in healthy infants. In our hospital (as in others) there were no planned observation periods of systematic recording of vital signs for infants after birth. A review of charts in our hospital had revealed that on the day of birth, information on the baby's clinical course was not continuously obtained or was totally lacking during the following periods:

1. The second stage of labor while preparations for delivery were being made.

2. The stay of the infant in the delivery room, from the time of his one-minute Apgar evaluation until his admission to the nursery. This time varied, lasting anywhere from 15 to 60 minutes after birth.

3. The initial hours in the nursery, from the time the baby was admitted and inspected by the nurse, until his examination by the physician. This time varied from 10 minutes to six hours after birth.

Thus, in our routine care of the fetus and the neonate, three "lost" or "limbo" periods occurred on the natal day – the day of highest neonatal morbidity and mortality.

First, we had to define a normal newborn infant. Since the words "normal" or "well" cannot, in a strict sense, be applied to infants who have received analgesics or anesthetics, even though indirectly through the placenta, we substituted the term, "standard baby." Four criteria were used for the "standard" classification: vaginal delivery, vertex presentation, birth weight of 2,500 grams or more, Apgar score of seven or higher.

With our criteria established, we began by following the infant from birth through the first hours of life.

FINDINGS

The First Period of Reactivity
The vigorous infant begins life with intense activity, which is characterized by

outbursts of diffuse, purposeless movements, alternating with brief periods of relative immobility. During this time, the respiration is rapid (the mean peak respiration rate is 82 breaths per minute occurring at one hour of age). Transient flaring of the alae nasi, retraction of the chest, and grunting are not unusual. Tachycardia is present (the mean peak heart rate of 180 beats per minute occurs at three minutes of age). The heart rate falls during the period of the most intense activity reaching an average of 120 to 140 beats per minute at approximately 30 minutes of age. Following this initial outburst, the infant becomes quiet and relatively unresponsive to either internal or external stimuli, at which time he becomes relaxed and may fall asleep. The average age when the first sleep begins is two hours, with this period lasting from a few minutes to two to four hours.

The Second Period of Reactivity
On awakening, the infant may be temporarily hyper-responsive to all stimuli. We have called this phase the second period of reactivity. The heart rate responds actively to stimulation, and there are swift changes in color. Frequently, the appearance of oral mucus is a major problem at this time, as it may be associated with gagging, swallowing, vomiting and, occasionally, choking.

This, the transition period in its entirety is similar to that of the post-operative patient in the recovery room. The infant must recover from the birth process as well as from the anesthesia or drug influences, or both, and, as any nurse knows well, recovery is not always uncomplicated. When the second period of reactivity is over, the infant is relatively stable; and we believe that he is well on his way to recovering from labor and delivery.

In the transitional care nursery, in addition to recording vital signs before and after feeding, research staff check the rooting, sucking, and swallowing reflexes. Even though these reflexes were present singly, many of the standard babies observed were unable initially to coordinate the sucking and swallowing reflexes and were prone to gag and regurgitate after feeding. (A postoperative patient is not fed routinely at 12 hours after surgery; he is fed when he recovers satisfactorily.) We have learned that every baby does not react the same way nor at the same time and that it is a good practice to offer the first feeding when the infant is relatively stable (after the second period of reactivity) and has good sucking and swallowing coordination.

Complicated Transition
The infant who begins extra-uterine life under adverse conditions has increased problems in recovery. Term infants (Apgar score of six or below and physiologically unresponsive infants) with low initial Apgar scores differ in their clinical course from the standard infant. Depressed infants (Apgar score of six or below and physiologically unresponsive infants) tend to have a low or falling

heart rate on delivery. The initial acceleration in heart rate is delayed, the period of rapid respiration is both delayed and prolonged, and the passage of meconium occurs at a later time. The infant of low birth weight likewise shows marked delays and exaggerations during transition. The second period of reactivity may occur after 12 or 18 hours of age, a factor which may be important in relation to planning the time of initial oral feeding. Infants whose mothers have been given premedication which tends to depress respiration may fail to show the initial period of rapid respiration, and bowel clearance may be late in onset.

Respiratory Problems

After birth, respiration may stop following the initial gasping and crying, and the infant's condition may deteriorate rapidly. This secondary apnea may follow too vigorous suction of the posterior pharynx. During the first hour, the infant may show intermittent retraction and grunting, and he is in danger of developing cyanosis and hypotonia, and real distress as a result of severe asphyxia. The baby should be handled little at this stage, and oxygen should be ready.

Cord Hemorrhage

Slight oozing from the umbilical vessels may occur between the second and sixth hour of age. It is frequently associated with crying or passage of meconium.

Mucus

The difficulties mucus can cause have already been discussed but may bear repeating — gagging, vomiting, breath holding, retracting the head, with choking and cyanosis, may occur in the second period of reactivity following the first sleep.

In summary, the nursery is only a halfway house between labor and delivery and the outside world. The potential of the infant and his ability to learn may be decided during fetal life and neonatal life — a period of rapid physiologic change.

APGAR SCORING

The Apgar scoring system to evaluate the condition of newborn infants was devised in 1952 by Virginia Apgar, then an anesthesiologist at Sloan Hospital for Women in New York City. Dr. Apgar reported several years later in the December 13, 1958 issue of the *Journal of the American Medical Association* that "60 seconds after the entire birth of the infant, irrespective of delivery of the placenta, represented the most severe depression after birth." In this scoring system, two points are assigned to each of five vital signs in the one-minute old infant: color, respiration, muscle tone, nasal irritability, and heart rate. "All infants with a score of 8, 9, or 10 are vigorous and have breathed within seconds of delivery." Dr. Apgar said that infants with a score of 4 or lower are limp, blue, and have not established respiration by one minute.

METHOD OF SCORING IN EVALUATION OF NEWBORN INFANT

SIGN	SCORE		
	0	1	2
Heart rate	Absent	Slow (<100)	>100
Respiratory effort	Absent	Weak cry; hypoventilation	Good: strong cry
Muscle tone	Limp	Some flexion of extremities	Well flexed
Reflex irritability (response of skin stimulation to feet)	No response	Some motion	Cry
Color	Blue: pale	Body pink; extremities blue	Completely pink

Briefly list the stages that the newborn must pass through to be ready for the world. When do these steps occur? Compare the transition period for the infant with that of the post operative patient.

When the admitting nursery nurse says, "he has an Apgar score of four or a score of nine" what does this mean to you, who must care for him during the first eight hours after birth or the third eight hours?

Why do the first 24 hours of life differ from the hours following?

List three types of potential problems that might occur during the first 12 to 18 hours of life.

16.

The First Year of Life

Gwendoline Bellam

As a nurse, how would you respond to the following parent comments about newborns and why?
". . . sleeps with his head on his left side all the time; won't that cause a misshapen head?"
". . . Mary spits up her milk almost as fast as she swallows it."
"Our new baby has a cold and he doesn't want his bottle."

He squirms, he kicks, he yells. Thus, seemingly under protest, another newborn is ushered into the outside world. He began life as a single cell, even smaller than the dot over the letter "i." But at birth he has two billion cells and is 35 hundred times the size of that dot. What a tremendous rate of growth this is.

Even more important than the changes that take place between conception and birth are those occurring during the first year of life. Development at this time is both rapid and exciting. Nurses aware of both the normal and abnormal – and the fine shades between – in the course of these 12 months have the foundation for appropriate intervention as indicated. Parents, too, would be spared many unnecessary worries and could take more delight in watching their child develop if they knew what to expect.

All the major organs are formed between the second and third months of intrauterine life. It will take several months, sometimes even years, of postnatal development, however, before these organs will be able to function as efficiently as they do in adult life. Similarly, as early as five months before birth, almost all the nerve cells a baby will ever possess are formed, and many are prepared to function in an orderly way.

Thus, we see a continuous and progressive process in effect from conception until senescence and death. It is, furthermore, an orderly process – one in which there is a direct relationship between each stage and the next one. This means that many experiences in early life are significant in determining physiologic and psychosocial functioning in later years. This should be clearly understood not only by the members of the various disciplines concerned with child and family welfare, but by parents themselves. For the nurse this knowledge is the keystone for her informed intervention.

During the embryonic stage, the human being is pretty much a parasite, completely dependent upon the mother for its very life. This dependency exists in varying degrees after, as well as before, birth. But because the external environment is so vastly different from the warmth, safety, and quietness of the intrauterine world, the infant's needs differ and become much more complex.

NEUROLOGIC DEVELOPMENT

The normal newborn is a reflex individual: nonthinking and, generally, nonpurposive. He functions at this reflex level for about the first six weeks of life, or until his forebrain is developed. Some of his reflex responses are demonstrated in his ability to root, suck, swallow, cough, gag, and sneeze. But he can "swallow up" just as easily as he can "swallow down," for his swallowing reflex is not strong at birth.

Development is intimately related to maturation of the nervous system. Thus, the persistence of reflexes for the first few months of life reflects the young infant's neurologic immaturity. No amount of encouragement or practice, for instance, can cause a child to walk until his nervous system is ready for it. Overambitious parents should realize this; otherwise they will frustrate both themselves and their child.

All reflexes are significant and can serve as helpful guidelines to developmental progress or the lack of it. The grasp, for example, is a strong but immature response occurring normally during the first few weeks of life. Just as strong a response is a baby's preference for lying with his head on one side, or turning his head to that side. There is no point in trying to change his head position, for he will just turn it back to the side of his preference, and he will persist in this for approximately the first six weeks of life. This is normal.

The Moro (startle) and tonic neck (fencing) reflexes, are normally present for about the first three or four months of life. Their absence at this time, however, or their persistence beyond it, indicates some neurologic deficiency. Persistence of the tonic neck reflex – a postural reflex – is one of the earlier manifestations of cerebral palsy.

Neurologic maturation goes hand in hand with the development of motor skills. Motor development proceeds in the cephalocaudal – from head to shoulders to abdomen, and so on — and the proximodistal — shoulder to fingertips, hips to toes — directions. This is as orderly a process as any of the other developmental sequences. The baby may pass through the various stages very rapidly, however, so the mother should be clued in as to what to watch for and expect, if she is to derive the fullest pleasure from watching her child grow and develop.

It will add to her satisfaction, too, if she understands that each new motor skill is a sign of the infant's growing mastery of self. Thus, the 16-week-old infant who moves his fingers and hands in front of his eyes is going through a fleeting developmental phase wherein he is learning about himself — touching, playing with, and seeing the various parts of his body. His pleasure in discovering that these hitherto fragmentory "objects" are all part of himself serves as his impetus for further investigation and discovery. Without this pleasurable ego response, he would fail to learn.

Those caring for him, though, need to realize that as his motor skills increase, so does the possibility of accidents. He can be expected to roll from back to side at approximately four months, roll over completely when he is about six months, and start creeping around the age of nine to ten months.

PHYSICAL GROWTH

During the first four to five months of life the infant gains approximately six to eight ounces a week, doubling his birth weight at about the end of this time. By the end of a year, his height is usually half again what it was at birth. Weight should be proportionate to height. The "overstuffed" baby of whom so many mothers are proud is not necessarily a healthy one. After this first year, the child's physical growth will proceed at a slower rate until he reaches puberty; then, physical growth again accelerates markedly.

This rapid growth during the first year, especially the first half of it, is reflected in the infant's food intake. As his growth rate begins to slow down, his appetite decreases, too, since his needs are not as great. This change in appetite is often a matter of concern to mothers if they are not prepared for it.

The infant's head circumference is usually about 13 inches at birth and will increase approximately 5 inches during the first 12 months. This rapid expansion is to accommodate the brain, which grows at a correspondingly rapid rate. At birth the brain is 25 percent its adult size. It increases 50 percent in size during the first year, and another 20 percent the second year. Obviously, prevention of head injury in this crucial period is important.

PHYSIOLOGIC DEVELOPMENT

Growth implies an increase in metabolism, and this leads to an increase in oxygen requirement. To meet this increased requirement, the infant's respiratory system is necessarily more active than that of the adult. In addition, his small physical size implies a short circulatory circuit, so that his pulse rate is also more rapid than in adulthood.

Because of the immature innervation of his intercostal muscles, the infant breathes with his abdominal muscles and diaphragm for approximately the first 18 months of this life. Thus, abdominal distention from any cause can impair respiratory function.

The chest of the young infant is cylindrical in shape and the thoracic cavity is small. All of this adds up to a very limited lung capacity, which explains the small infant's acute response to a respiratory infection that an older child would react to only minimally. In addition, the infant can breathe only through his nose for the first four to five weeks of life. If his nares become blocked by accumulated secretions, this will add to his respiratory distress. Under these circumstances, he may also reject his feedings since he is using all his available energy to maintain his respiratory functioning.

The infant's daily fluid turnover is 15 percent of his total body weight as compared to the adult's turnover of 9 percent. Some aspects of kidney development are not complete until the child is two years of age. In the neonatal period, insensible water loss from skin and lungs is larger in proportion to body weight than at any other period of life. A highly humidified atmosphere decreases this insensible water loss, but other circumstances will determine when or if the infant should be placed in such an atmosphere.

The endocrine system is the least ready of all body systems for extrauterine activities. This explains the newborn's frequently irregular and unstable temperature, because the thyroid and adrenal glands play important roles in stabilizing body temperature. Spontaneous variations of from $1°-2°F$. are common during the first year of life.

With each Fahrenheit degree of temperature increase, there is a 7.2 percent increase in metabolism. This implies a need for increased fluid intake to facilitate excretion of the end products of this stepped-up metabolism, as well as to compensate for the fluids lost through the increased respiratory activity precipitated by the elevated temperature. Of course, the pulmonary system is not the only one to undergo physiologic stress as a result of a temperature elevation.

PSYCHOSOCIAL DEVELOPMENT

The real catalyst for physical development is the infant's psychosocial development, which plays a significant role in triggering the hoped-for responses in his other areas of growth. This psychosocial development is completely dependent upon the infant's interpersonal relationships with his mother or mother supplement; the groundwork for such relationships is first established during the mother's own childhood, and begins with her infant immediately after his birth.

To be effective, the relationship must be a continuing one. If interruptions are unavoidable, they should not be prolonged ones since it is through the consistent ministrations of his mother or mother supplement that the infant's basic needs are met.

Initially, he is very demanding — "he wants what he wants when he wants it." But, as his demands are consistently and lovingly met, he begins to realize that the person responsible for the giving is a person whom he can trust. As this trust and sense of well-being develop, the child's demands decrease. He is able to wait — the beginning of a sense of self and of independence!

A very important part of this process is any mother-child activity involving physical handling of the child. The tactile sense is already highly developed at birth, and touch and close physical contact — essential ingredients of mothering — can communicate security and trust to the infant and give him the inner strength to cope with new experiences.

Such mothering is an emotional experience and a skill that the new mother must learn. It doesn't always follow automatically upon the birth of the infant. It may take some mothers weeks or even months to achieve a state of equilibrium in this new role. Help from the nurse in this respect is nearly always welcomed.

Growth is a continuing and exciting process. Although it proceeds in an orderly fashion, development in any one area is closely related to and influenced by development in other areas. The nurse who understands this and is familiar with the normal processes of growth and development is in a position to determine whether or not an infant is progressing at a normal rate and manner, to take prompt and appropriate action when she observes the abnormal, and to give thoughtful and scientifically based nursing care. And, to the degree that the nurse shares this information with the mother, she contributes to the infant's well-being and the mother's sense of security during the all-important first year of life.

How do you react to the statement that a baby is a parasite and that this dependency continues in varying degrees after birth?

What does it mean to be a "reflex individual," and how does this affect nursing care for the first six weeks of life?

What important factors should be explained about neurologic development and the child with overambitious parents?

How might growth and development differ for an infant who is very active from that of one who is very docile in relation to fluid intake and mothering?

List six facts included in this article that would be appropriate for discussion with a new mother during her postpartum stay in the hospital.

17.
Play PRN in Pediatric Nursing

Jacqueline Hott

It may seem strange to devote a particular section to "play."
What seems to be a normal and established part of everyday
life may disappear in a crisp, sterile, hospital situation. Think
about your own feelings as an efficient, capable nurse playing
with a little patient instead of quickly carrying out your skilled
procedures. Perhaps after reading this article you will recognize
play as a skill to be learned and practiced.

Sixty years ago fun was suspect in child training and was regarded as inappropriate and frivolous in patient care. Playing with the baby was considered dangerous, and playing with the child in the hospital was thought to be excessively stimulating and deleterious with overtones of erotic excitement. This "fun taboo" was a remnant of our Puritanical culture; one felt guilty about enjoying oneself, and to have fun while working was tantamount to insincerity and deception.

Play in the hospital, on an organized basis, was introduced in 1930, when the Children's Memorial Hospital in Chicago in an attempt to give its patients experiences considered compatible with childhood, initiated a full-time program of play as an essential part of its treatment of children. To acquaint the nursing personnel and the volunteer play leaders with the many types of play which children enjoy and to give them practice in the activities suited to the hospital situation, a course in play was given as part of a study in human relationships. In twenty correlated lectures and demonstrations various aspects of play were presented: play as entertainment, as an aid to treatment, as a means of understanding the child's behavior and promoting his mental health, and as an aid to his total development.

Nonetheless, the course in play, along with their experiences on the wards, changed the attitudes of many of the nurses toward play, toward children as patients, and toward their work as nurses in pediatrics. My observations on a large pediatric service revealed that nurses seemed to avoid the playroom, and play leaders expressed the feeling that nurses have more important things to do. The nurses, when asked why they did not play in the playroom with their patients said, "That's the play lady's job" or, "We don't get paid to play."

It is important that the nurse *be aware of the importance of play as a nursing care activity.* For it is the nurse's role to focus on the child rather than on his sickness. Parents and nurses need to be released from the inhibiting effects of focusing their attention on disabilities and from the block which makes them assume that the child with impaired hearing, for example, would need a different kind of plaything from that used by the child with normal hearing. As nurses acquire more insight into the developmental and psychological needs of children, they will perceive the importance of a hospital setting which is more homelike and where they, as mother substitutes, are warm, friendly, and understanding. This awareness is part of the recognition that "hospitalitis" is not eliminated by nursing that is merely technically efficient. The only way to ensure adequate care of a child in the hospital is to create an emotional bond between the adult nurse and her young patient so that nursing is fused with mothering. This is the essence of a "therapeutic community" in the hospital, where play must be part of the total service and all the people working with each child must be concerned with more than just the child's physical needs. To implement the concept of the therapeutic community greater acceptance of play as therapy, based upon an understanding of the philosophy of play, should be promoted among nurses who work with children.

The play leader's records showed that most of the nursing personnel who were taking the course, either as affiliating students in pediatric nursing or as graduate nurses, had had limited experience of any sort with children. Accustomed as they were to thinking of play as amusement and having had their tutelage in hospitals which were still representative of the American Puritan heritage, they found the new ideas about play alien.

Their training in nursing had stressed the physical care of the acutely ill child. Their own play experience and attitudes had been colored by the competitive types of play that high schools and colleges offer, such as basketball, hockey, tennis, archery, and swimming, most of which were unsuitable for bed-bound or ambulatory convalescent children. Many of them felt that play was just a convenient means of keeping the children quiet. It was not easy for them to accept spontaneity, initiative, and attention to human relationships as essentials in employing play as a therapeutic tool.

THEORIES OF PLAY

Of special importance to the nurse are the theories that relate to the value of play in various developmental stages. Infants and children vary in their modes of response to play situations, so that sensory stimulation for the infant and verbal stimulation for the older child must be evaluated and interpreted on a level that is psychologically meaningful for each. It begins before it is noticed as play and consists of the exploration or repetition of sensual perceptions, kinesthetic sensations, or vocalizations. The nurse, aware of this developmental phase, plays with the infant as she feeds him, bathes him, and dresses him, talking, singing, moving her head up and down, smiling, stroking the infant, and letting him explore her face and fingers with his own. These are the baby's first "geography lessons," and the "topographical knowledge" acquired in such interplay is a guide for his first orientation to the world. This is the kind of play most easily duplicated by the mother when she is made aware of its value.

The *microsphere* is the small world of manageable toys with which the child first tries to master the world of "things"; failure to achieve such mastery, caused by illness or neglect, results in a continuation of the autospheric defenses of daydreaming, thumbsucking, and masturbating. At nursery school age, play becomes a world of the *macrosphere,* which the child shares with others before going on to the next stage of mastery. There are the play activities of an imaginative, dramatic character in which children use available *objects* – blocks, chairs, or toys – as instruments in the play schema. In the other type of play the child tries to rehearse make-believe activities, transforming available materials into tools in order to enter the adult world for a time. Thus, the discarded plastic 10 cc. syringe becomes a tool which can be used in playing nurse or doctor and for inflicting upon the nurse, the child's "patient," some of the pain of his own world. The child can withdraw whenever he is bored or frustrated by the difficult requirements of this adult world.

When the nurse participates in this make-believe, she reassures the child that his play is valid and meaningful, gives him strength to cope with it, and shows him that he has adult approval to go on striving for mastery in the play situation. For this kind of communication participation in play is more effective than is language. Recently I was a "passenger" on a "bus" constructed by patients in the hospital playroom out of every available chair in the room. Part of the children's delight came from having the nurse, an adult, take part in this drama, thereby enhancing its meaning.

For the child, the name and the thing, fantasy and reality, lying and telling the truth are not clearly separated. Certain types of substitution are possible only in a play situation in which objects do not have the fixed characterization that they do in a serious situation. In the serious situation, the child usually refuses the play substitute, and conversely, the child in the play situation will often refuse a real action as a substitute for the play action. The nurse will see this clearly when observing that the child who wants the real (used) hypodermic syringe, because of its serious experiential meaning to him, will not be satisfied with the toy one from the play-doctor set, but that the child who is playing patient and getting shots will not want to substitute the real injection for the play one.

The nurse may be meeting inner goals by caring for the critically ill child postoperatively, when the child is completely dependent upon her, whereas inner goals may not be met by playing peek-a-boo or "Where is thumbkin?" with the convalescing child. What the nurse does not understand is that the recuperating child may be just as dependent upon her for play as part of essential nursing care.

PLAY THERAPY

In developing an understanding of philosophy of play in pediatric nursing, the professional nurse must use this knowledge constructively by making play important in her nursing practice. For, in addition to the benefits from play which accrue to any child, play offers special value to the child who is hospitalized. Proper play can bring relaxation and induce the rest necessary in the care and treatment of the sick child.

Many hospitalized children tend to receive passively and without question the needles, operations, examinations, and medications that nurses and doctors deem best for them. This passive conformity leaves small possibility for the patient to participate actively within his environment. The nurse can provide through play some of the vocal and physical outlets the child needs for expression of his feelings as well as his urge to be productive.

During hospitalization, children are exposed to a variety of new and unfamiliar people, routines, procedures, sounds, and smells, but although these stimuli may be very high at certain times, they are almost nonexistent at other times.

Play therapy is directed at helping the hospitalized child to make a better adjustment to the hospital, to himself and his illness, and to life in general; thus, it contributes to his social and emotional well-being.

The key person in the life of the hospitalized child is the nurse who, even when there is a play lady, must provide many hours of play. She does not have to wait for a scheduled play period, just as a mother does not rigidly assign a time of day as a play period for her to share with her child outside of the day's routine. The nurse can start play while she is giving bedside care by telling simple stories to the individual child or a group of children. Storytelling, whether imaginative or anecdotal, can be part of every day's care. To the child who cannot understand or respond to a story, a nurse can repeat nursery rhymes, finger-plays, or snatches of poetry and song, and even commercial jingles. Many of the youngest children respond to conversation about favorite television personalities, and familiarity with the cartoon shows and the characters and methods of "Sesame Street" should be part of a pediatric nurse's background knowledge.

The nurse must be willing to allow the child considerable freedom in his use of water, and be ready to spend extra time with him during his bath. Boats, bubble bath, wash cloths, sponge objects, and other toys are most helpful in stimulating water play. For example, to the cerebral palsied child blowing soap bubbles across the basin is a play way to practice the techniques he must learn as a requisite to speech improvement. For the child who needs to strengthen his arm muscles, filling and squeezing a bath sponge is akin to the technique a big league pitcher uses when he squeezes a rubber ball to increase his muscular strength and control. When the young child bathes his doll the nurse frequently has an opportunity to elicit his verbalization about anxieties concerning his own body image.

It is important that the nurse spend time with the children in the playroom. It is equally important that she honor the "sanctity and neutrality" of the playroom. It is not the place for giving medication or introducing intrusive or painful procedures; it represents the child's "territorial imperative." It should be a place for unfolding wings, not clipping them. In even the most child-centered ward arrangement it is the nurse who gives the commands. (Turn. Move. Sit Up. Lie down. Sit on the potty. It's time to take your temperature, open your mouth.) In the playroom the child becomes the most important person and is in command of the situation. No one nags or suggests or goads him on or pries into his private world. As Jeffrey said, "I'm going to miss all this when I go home. It's like a palace in the playroom. I can do anything I want and play anything I want to play."

It is a nursing responsibility to recognize the importance of play as a way of coping with life competently. Some adults find their play in their work; others find love in their work. For the developing child, play *is* his work; for the sick child in the hospital, convalescing signals a resumption of this work.

A physically and emotionally well child becomes dissatisfied unless he has a sense of being useful and of making things and making them well and perfectly. He wants to win recognition by producing things and to bring a productive situation to completion. Once a project is begun, it is important that the child try to finish it in the playroom or on the bedtable. Therefore, perfection must be oriented to the child's ability, not the nurse's; the child should not be involved in a long, taxing, or frustrating endeavor that is beyond his capabilities. It is difficult for the nurse to restrain herself from filling in the puzzle pieces or finishing off the doll's dress or putting the final touches on a painting or a sketch. Do remnants of her own sense of industry interfere with the nurse's play with the child? Does she still feel, perhaps, that making things "well and perfectly," like bed corners, nurses' notes, and treatment trays, are the "useful" things and that play does not give her this recognition?

To the child who has been sick for a long time, or is in a body cast, or is in isolation, loneliness and inactivity are painfully familiar. If active play is impossible or really dangerous to the child's progress toward health, he may come to feel that any activity is dangerous. An acute helplessness may ensue, especially if he is immobilized or isolated. In such instances, the need to entertain and stimulate the child is especially urgent.

The child who is in isolation and who cannot leave his room even on a stretcher or in a wheelchair needs to have an environment which will decrease his feeling of physical isolation. Mirrors are helpful allies here, and the child should be helped to adjust them so that they reflect as much activity as possible. A repertoire of finger-play games, songs, stories, and other individualized skills of the experienced nurse are a must for this child.

To many nurses and parents, television-viewing is considered a form of play, and the pros and cons of its use in the hospital must be considered. Hospitalization is therefore not necessarily the time to wean the child away from television, particularly if these habitual programs are satisfying and "just like home." The child's needs should determine how he uses television, and the question becomes the quality of the program, not the length of time spent viewing. The alert nurse can use the break for the commercial (unless the commercial is better than the program!) for special treatments that must be carried out frequently during the day. For example, for the child convalescing from surgery, the nurse and the child can plan together that at the next break the catheter will be irrigated, or another glass of juice will be taken, or deep-breathing or coughing will be done in rhythm to the commercial jingle.

When the nurse understands the functions of play in the hospital, she will be able to guide parents who oversupply their sick child with toys; she will know how to hold back something special for that "rainy" day. The rainy day might be when the mother has been delayed in visiting· or when a treatment particularly frightening or painful is to be given. Whenever possible, the mother's guidance about special games or songs which are part of the child's daily routine should be sought. The mother's response that no special play themes exist and that she "never has time or fools around like that" should not deter the nurse from establishing a pattern of play which will sustain the child during his hospitalization and help him to master the deeper anxieties caused by separation. Rather, it provides an opportunity for the nurse to cooperate with the mother who does not know how to give of herself in play and to show her that giving her child attention does not necessarily mean "spoiling" him.

It is conceivable that almost every nurse in pediatrics at some time in her life has had the experience of being in a strange place where she was unknown and somewhat unsure of what would be happening. Like the stranger in a foreign country who suddenly hears his own language, the child reaches out to play in anticipation of friendship in a bewildering and frightening situation. When the child shares play with the nurse he discovers a sensitive and responsive human being. Play, as an integral part of pediatric nursing, will help us to put the pieces together.

Why is it important for an adult to participate in some of the child's play?

How do you feel about caring for children during the critical and convalescent stages of illness? What appeals to you most and why?

List and describe the purposes and advantages of play as listed in this article. Try the techniques and evaluate your feelings and the child's reactions.

18.
Immobilized Youth

Florence G. Blake

If you had a choice, would you care for a two-year-old, a nine-year-old, or a fifteen-year-old who is immobilized in traction for six weeks or longer? Why? How would you cope or help them cope with the frustrations of being unable to be up and about? What is supportive care?

Personnel in hospitals are often less confident of their ability to support school-agers and adolescents than they are to provide understanding care for little children. Expression of feeling in older children is difficult for many personnel to bear; it frightens them and arouses feelings of helplessness and worry. Thus, they often perceive supportive nursing care of older children as more difficult than it really is.

Another reason the care of older children and adolescents may be distressing for hospital personnel is the discrepancy which exists between their own perceptions, interests, and goals and those of their patients. Doctors and other personnel perceive hospitals as institutions of healing, but from most children's point of view, hospitals are not anything as benevolent as that. The doctor's goal — cure, or rehabilitation, or both — is often remote, while children's goals center on their current needs for pleasure and growing up.

Understanding the new tasks, frustrations, and feelings that confront school-agers and young adolescents immobilized for medical treatments is the basis of confidence in one's ability to support school-agers and adolescents when they lose control of their feelings or are in a panic lest they might.

Emotional support in stressful situations will make it less common to observe in the school-age and adolescent populations in hospitals, a high incidence of depression, stoicisms, disinterest in schoolwork, apathetic responses to the recreational program, and resistance to the staff's efforts to guide them in learning to protect their health and to participate actively in the coping and rehabilitation process.

PURPOSES OF MOTILITY

The motor phase of psychosocial development reaches its peak of intensity between the second and tenth year of life and continues to a lesser degree into late adolescence. The infant's motor system helps him to discover the reality of separateness from his mother. It helps him to gain control of many of his impulses. It aids him in testing reality and in reducing his fear of the world beyond his home which, when accomplished, provides new kinds of stimulation, motivation to learn, and knowledge for problem solving. Motor activity also provides constructive outlets for feelings, tension, and aggression.

The achievement of motor skills is an important factor in gaining control over feelings of helplessness and inferiority and enhances the child's opportunities for social relationships with peers. Furthermore, the capacity to move quickly and ably serves a protective function; it makes it possible to fight an aggressor or to take flight from danger.

Thus, it is plain to see how an intact motor system and guidance to use it in socially acceptable ways contributes to the development of a healthy self- and body-image. It is also easy to see how defects in the motor system, inhibitions in using his powers of motility, or prolonged frustration from periods of immobilization during the formative years of a child's life can block psychosocial development and/or cause distortions in his self- and body-image.

PSYCHOSOCIAL EFFECTS

Life in the hospital superimposes another set of problems on those the young person was struggling with at home and in school before admission. When he is admitted to the hospital the energy the young person used to cope with the developmental crisis usual for his age becomes absorbed in his struggle to deal with the demands of a new environment.

Unless the young person learns quickly that he can trust the staff to prepare him for impending painful procedures and to provide support during these procedures, he will expend his precious energy in keeping his frightening feelings under rigid control, or act them out in ways which are distressful not only to him but to the staff as well.

Loss of control of strong feelings with temper outbursts, tears, or overt demonstration of fear is ego-alien to most young people. It leads to a guilty conscience and loss of self-esteem unless there is someone close by who understands and can help the young person know he does not need to expect himself to be a stoic all the time when he is confined in bed, a cast, or on a treatment table. This will help him to know that she wants to help him to talk over his problems with her.

There are many reasons immobilization is a most depriving and threatening part of hospitalization for young people. It frustrates their natural urge for motility and their need for the many pleasures derived from it. The walls of the hospital in and of themselves are perceived as restraints by young people. They cut them off from association with those persons they need the most—parents, siblings, friends—to master natural developmental tasks. They prevent them from going into parts of the world they have already mastered and from which they obtained a great deal of pleasure. Hospital walls confine them in small areas that prevent them from conquering their fear of unknown parts of the institution. They also make it difficult for them to select their friends and caretakers and to get the kinds of stimulation and activity they need to reduce boredom. Equally trying for many young people is deprivation of opportunities for solitude when they need it.

When the young person goes out of bounds because of loneliness, sensory deprivation, or intolerable tension from other frustrations or worries, scoldings or penalties increase his burdens. They not only reinforce unacceptable behavior, but also increase the level of his tension. Under these circumstances, the punished young person often feels misunderstood. He will probably become more needful of motor activity to cope constructively with his aggression as well.

When young persons must be confined to bed in a body sling or cast or be immobilized in traction without time to mobilize their resources to prepare themselves to participate in this kind of treatment, marked rise in anxiety can be anticipated. When immobilizing equipment restricts patterns of behavior used in the past to relieve frustration and discharge aggression, the young person's discomfort from anxiety will be intensified. Even when the rationale for treatment has been shared with the young person and he is able to involve himself in preparation for it, he will be fearful of the unknown and therefore in a state of emotional disequilibrium until he acquires constructive coping devices to deal with the new and difficult tasks which will undoubtedly confront him.

NURSING INTERVENTION

One characteristic of crises of particular importance in providing nursing care is that though crises present dangers, they also provide opportunities for growth in adaptive capacity. Wise, carefully planned support during the immobilizing event and in the period thereafter can help the young person attain a higher level of mental health than he had achieved before the onset of the threatening event.

Supportive nursing intervention entails a knowledge of the doctor's goals and plan of care and competence in the provision of physical care to provide comfort and conserve the patient's energy for healing and problem solving. It also entails careful study of the young person while he is being immobilized and in the period immediately thereafter.

The young person's parents also will need help in dealing with their feelings about their offspring's need for immobilization. They will welcome the chance to assist in designing and implementing an initial plan of care.

Ted and Jim were typical examples of adolescents suffering the frustrations of immobilization. Jim was nearly 13 years of age and in a cast following a spinal fusion to prevent further scoliosis. Ted, an obese 15-year-old, had had one operation on his foot and was facing another.

One evening Ted stalked aggressively up to the desk, waved a leather-craft metal chisel in front of the nurse's face and growled: "Don't let this get into our room again or I'll kill him." Ted's facial expression, tone of voice, gestures, and words denoted fury. Because this behavior signaled a call for help, I trailed Ted to his room at the far end of the corridor. For a minute I was frightened! I didn't know Ted, and had had only one or two brief contacts with Jim. Nor did I know what had provoked Ted's fury. However, he was in panic lest he lose control of his aggression, and I knew from experience, that nothing helps young people under these circumstances as much as discovering that others are not as frightened of their impulses as they are; that the causes of their frustration are understandable to others, and that adults have faith in their power to help themselves regain emotional equilibrium. Therefore, my goals were to help these young people feel understood rather than guilty, and to help them mobilize resources which would increase control over their aggression.

Once inside the room Ted got into a wheelchair and wheeled himself back and forth. I situated myself comfortably on an easy chair in the room. In less than a minute Ted and Jim, seemingly oblivious to my presence, fought each other with words.

Jim: I wasn't going to kill you, Ted. How else could I defend myself? You pulled my hair. And you know I can't get out of this cast.

Ted: Well, I had my foot operated on. They're going to fix my shoulder next. I talked to my psychiatrist today. I got lots of things straightened out. I was wrong on lots of things. My mother beat me. I can't stand dominating women. (There was a minute or two of silence.) You know, I thought coming into the hospital would be fun. But damn it. It isn't! (Ted turned his head and met my eyes.)

F.B.: No, life in the hospital isn't fun. I'll bet you fellows feel like caged lions. You must be as bored and frustrated as you can be.

Ted: You're telling me! I'll say I am. I need a gym. I need to work this out. I'm sick and tired of this room.

F.B.: When you're caged up together 24 hours a day, you get sick and tired of each other and all of the nurses. Perhaps you're even furious with each other, too.

Jim: You're telling me? But, honestly, nurse, I wasn't going to kill him.

F.B.: Of course, you weren't. You can control yourself.

Jim: You should have heard what he called an aide last night.

Ted: I just used the worst word I could think of. There are some times that I hate women. I'm in a reform school.

Ted's conversation about the reform school stimulated Jim to talk about guns and the experiences he had had in hunting. Temporarily, he had taken flight into fantasy which seemed to revive pleasant memories and perhaps even made him feel freer from restrictions than he had a few minutes before. Ted looked as if he, too, were enjoying a temporary escape from boredom. Then Ted said, "I've got a gun, too. We used to shoot at targets in the Milwaukee Park until the cops got after us." The boys had found a common interest and even expressed it verbally: they were already feeling more friendly to each other.

Jim added, "You should see what the kids at home do. They throw rocks at the school, get in through the windows and bust up the blackboards." To convey my interest and help Jim relieve his tension with talking, I said, "I wonder why they do that. What do you think?"

Jim replied, "You don't think up things like that when you're alone, but when you're with a gang you egg each other on. If you don't join the crowd, you're chicken. I guess it's better to do it than to be alone."

Then after a minute or two of thought, Jim demonstrated another personality strength. He said, "I sort of think I could find other kids to play with. I really don't want to get mixed up with them. But then . . . gosh you're chicken." To communicate empathy, I said, "And being chicken hurts." His response was immediate, "But it doesn't hurt as much as being caught."

Later in the conversation, Jim said, "I want to be a pilot but I know they'll never take me in the Air Force with this back. Maybe I can get into aeronautics."

His words told me something about his fantasies, his goals, and his ability to face reality. (Immobilized youngsters often have fantasies which imaginatively take them into wide open spaces with fewer barriers to freedom than in the hospital.) To help Jim know that he was understood, I responded with: "Right now, you'd like to do most anything but be cooped up in that cast."

Ted: Can't you get the doctors to order physiotherapy for me? I've got to get a work out. Then I could behave better. All the recreation around here is for six-year-old kids. There's nothing here for us.

I thought he had a good point and suggested that he ask his psychiatrist to order some exercise for him in the physical therapy department.

In a few minutes both boys acted as if they were more at ease. They seemed to detect each other's longing for an interested listener. To help them plan some activity for the evening hours, I asked if some card games would lessen their boredom, but the idea did not appeal to them. They both let off some steam about being "blastedly bored." Then Ted decided to write some letters and Jim thought he would do the same.

As I left to find the needed paper and envelopes, I said, "It will take me a while to find some but I will be back with them."

On my return, Ted asked for the cardboard off the writing pad. Later, I noticed a sign on the door with WOMEN printed on it in large black letters. Not quite sure what it meant, I said, "I wouldn't think you fellows would want this sign on your door." Ted responded quickly, "We want women to come in here." "Then why don't you tell them exactly that? You'd get better results if you did," I said. Jim responded with a smile and said, "Gosh, thanks. You know you've helped us a lot." Ted grabbed the marking pencil and triumphantly changed the sign to: WOMEN WELCOME.

It was a far cry from the look of fury and the brandished chisel.

Discuss being in the hospital through the eyes of an adult and a teenager. How can an immobilized person get away from a threatening situation? How can you help? How would you cope if your hospitalized teenager cries? Doesn't cry? Has angry outbursts? Is stoic?

Now that you have read about Ted and Jim, think about your own feelings as a person and how this would affect your supportive care as a nurse. Could you listen and react without judgment?

What five behavior problems might be prevented by giving children emotional support during stressful periods?

Give some specific examples of problems and support.

19.

How Children Perceive Pain

Nancy V. Schultz

The following selection discusses pain as perceived by children ten and eleven. Why do nurses need to know how children perceive pain and what can they do for them?

One person may accept pain almost gratefully, as punishment for misdeeds; another, hysterically, beyond comprehension; and someone else, happily, glad to be alive. Children often experience pain fearfully, not understanding what is happening to them. Regardless of how it is experienced, pain causes change.

Pain alters the person feeling it—physiologically, (via nerve pathways) by changing one's posture, gait, heart rate, or blood pressure; or psychologically and emotionally by causing restlessness, anxiety, hostility, anger, anguish, or despair. Whatever its degree, pain always causes change, change causes stress, and stress increases pain. Thus a vicious circle evolves and is perpetuated. Somewhere, somehow, this circle must be broken.

Rather than concentrate exclusively on the family's coping mechanisms or the theories about pain, nurses should also apply principles of growth and development—that is, the behavior and characteristics of people at various age-stages of development. It was for this reason—to improve my nursing care of children—that I elected to learn more about the attitudes and perception of pain of ten- and eleven-year-old children and relate that information to normal growth and development.

My reason then, for conducting a survey of their perception of pain was to understand some of the commonalities in the way children in the same age-stage of development have experienced it or perceived it.

HOW, NOT WHY

I wanted to find out *how* children at a fixed age-stage of development view pain, rather than *why* they react to it as they do. I believed that if we could learn, before a child is admitted to a hospital, how he might react to pain just because he *is* three, five, eight, or ten, we could begin to give him support immediately and with more understanding.

THE STUDY

The study group consisted of 74 ten and eleven-year-old boys and girls.

Since I could not interview each child, I constructed a list of questions I thought them capable of answering. The only vital statistics I asked for were age and sex and they were unsigned.

1. Have you ever been in the hospital?

2. Why were you in the hospital?

3. List three things that have happened to you that made you feel pain.

4. Underline no more than *two* of the following: When I have pain I feel afraid, brave, nervous, like crying but I don't, like crying and I do.

5. What does pain mean to you? Write down everything that comes to your mind about pain.

The first two questions were asked mainly to secure data for use in future study; there may be a relationship between a child's perception of pain and his reaction to it if he has been hospitalized in the past. His perception may be hazy if he has blocked a bad experience, or clearer if he was successfully helped to cope with it. This topic requires much more study than I could give it in this survey.

The mere contrasts in choices picked by the children, for example, *brave* and *afraid, brave* and *won't cry, afraid/nervous* and *want to cry but won't*, should show us the conflict these children are in when experiencing pain. This in itself is worth intervention and understanding.

FEAR INCREASES PAIN

Fear of death is one aspect of the perception of pain that ten- and eleven-year-old children experience. It may be increased when the child is hospitalized, and such fear probably increases pain. Because this age group fears physical harm, their reaction is based more on their fear than on the pain experienced. In answer to the question: What does pain mean to you? Some of the replies were: "It hurts. It hurts inside." "I feel like screaming." "The doctor." "I think I'm going to die." "Getting shots. Getting injections." "It hurts so much it kills ya." "Like a hammer beating into me." "When something hurts real bad you get in shock." "I think it's serious but it never is."

It's helpful to know that their reaction to pain and fear of bodily damage are exaggerated, so that we do not either medicate these children unnecessarily, or ignore them because we feel they're being "babies" and making a "big deal" about nothing. Rather, we should realize that this is normal behavior for this age group, and try to group them with children their own age so they can complain to each other and share experiences.

Also, we need to spend time listening and reassuring them because their pain and fear are real. In light of the responses given, it would appear that some of our palliative measures—injections for pain, for example—are likely to cause more suffering and fear than the original pain. Oral medications would be wiser to use at these times.

Fear has many facets, as can be seen from some of the responses that were more abstract and dealt with pain and fear on another level. I was surprised at the following descriptions of pain that I think are justifiably critical of the stereotypes many of us have of ten- and eleven-year-olds. Pain is:

Being nervous (girl, ten years old).
Not growing up healthy (boy, eleven years old).
Being afraid (boy, eleven years old).
When you scream for help and nobody comes (girl, eleven
years old; had been hospitalized).
Going through the hospital with everyone looking at you
(boy, ten years old).
When something hurts you and you can't get help (girl,
eleven years old; had been hospitalized).

These statements contain implications for nursing intervention. How many times have we heard a child this age call for a nurse and be told to wait till the nurse stopped a toddler's crying, or finished her charting. It never before hit me so forcefully that these children would feel so abandoned. After counting responses and finding that 64 out of 74 children connected pain with being afraid or nervous, I would say that "fear is pain."

ANXIETY AND ANGER

Some of the children managed to put this elusive feeling of anxiety in relation to pain into words in stating pain is:

Something you have no control of.

You think it will never end.
Something that hurts and you can't stop it.
When you get nervous, you sweat, and feel tense; moaning.

What better source of anxiety than something you can't control! The mere fact that in their struggle for independence these children have to deal with something they cannot control is a problem in itself, without the added distress of physical pain. They practically tell us they can't help themselves, so it's clear that intervention is necessary. In light of their dependence-independence struggle, we can best intervene by helping them to help themselves control their pain. When their pain is lessened, their independence will be strengthened.

How we help each child will, of course, depend on the patient, and this, in turn, will depend on how the nurse uses her knowledge of his life style, of his parents' reactions to pain, and of how he has coped with pain in the past.

They are very "school conscious" and worry about poor grades and failing. Authorities on growth and development point this out, but how often do we meet this need when the child is in the hospital? In agreement with this need, some children said they viewed pain as, "getting a failing mark," "getting a bad report card."

If such statements identify situations that are viewed as pain or as being painful, it becomes our responsibility to help the child faced with this reaction. The recognition that such situations can be painful will give us a clue as to why the hospitalized child is sometimes destructive, belligerent, and hostile. When we realize that children this age might be angry at themselves for being ill, perhaps we can cease being punitive and begin to be more understanding. This alone, by lessening some of the anger and anxiety, will mitigate their painful experience. Thus we see—once again—that to a 10- or 11-year-old child, pain is not always the result of physical injury.

DRIVE AND ENERGY

One 11-year-old boy said, "The worst thing about pain is that you can't play football or any other kind of sport"; and a 10-year-old boy wrote, "When I broke my arm I worried that I wouldn't be able to pitch again." This says a lot. Often children view pain as a hindrance to their wants and needs, as well as a physical or psychological trauma. This is another facet of pain perception that an understanding of normal growth and development can help us to deal with.

Obviously, we can't get a game of football going in the playroom, but we can refrain from chastising children who get restless and mischievous in the hospital setting. We can do such positive things as allowing older children roommates who are their own age. Peer companionship is much needed by the mid-childhood group.

Middle childhood is a critical period during which conscience develops at a rapid rate. Some of the children viewed pain from a purely psychological point of view, thus showing the beginning of the development of mature levels of thinking. The children who took this view were all eleven years old, whereas most of the ten-year-olds discussed or described pain in physical terms. Both of these outlooks were "normal" for the children's ages, with those eleven showing increasing awareness of a more elusive type of pain—that caused by injury to one's feelings. Some of these responses regarding pain were:

If you do something wrong you feel bad.
Getting scolded.
When someone you love does something to hurt you.

Implications for nursing intervention for the relief of pain in this context are obvious. All that is required of us is that our attitudes be warm, accepting, and nonjudgmental, and that we treat the children like the feeling, thinking, persons they are. We must remember that children have feelings that can cause them pain or add to it. What is required of us is little more than practicing the golden rule. It may not always be easy to do, but it is important both to the children and to ourselves that we do it. We must be careful not to make judgments or create stereotypes, and we must be careful not to inflict pain through methods we use to alleviate it.

CONCLUSIONS

One theme emerges from this presentation—the nurse who would understand a child's reaction to pain must constantly look at the total, everchanging child in relation to his pain. This is how it must be if we would truly see a child as an open system, constantly interacting with his environment.

As we view the life processes of man, we see how the constant interaction between man and his environment is constantly changing him and being changed by him. Since I believe that change causes stress, that stress causes or can be caused by pain, and that pain causes or can be caused by change, I also believe that nurses must begin to view the normal processes a child goes through as the painful experiences that the child perceives them to be.

Pain isn't just a broken leg, or an injection; it is also growing, changing, being scolded, failing in school, and not having visitors. If we are to be truly helpful in alleviating a child's pain, we must first understand how he perceives pain and, second, we must learn to anticipate what might be a painful experience to a child of a certain age and take measures either to prevent or lessen it.

How would you answer the five questions the author used in her survey? Think back to an earlier pain felt at a certain age and try to remember your feelings.

Try the questions out on children of different ages and apply yourself to planning care as a result of their answers.

If you, as a nursing student, asked some pediatric patients these questions (and listened to and recorded their answers), what would you then do with the information? What if you were doing it as a staff nurse? Would your actions differ and, if so, why?

You may be more aware now of how little we really know about this young age group. Why do you think there is so little real information?

THE OLD

20.
Why Old People Fall

Mieczyslaw Peszczynski

*As you prepare to assist patients to ambulate, you must think
about what age and learning has to do with how a person
walks. Visualize these four different age groups walking (if
you can't do this, sit in a park or stand on a street corner and
observe): a toddler, a teenager, an adult, and an aged person.*

Older persons fall more frequently than younger ones do. All of us are aware of
this. We caution older persons to be careful and to reduce hazards in their
environment that may contribute to falls.

Most of us walk without thinking much about it, but how do we do it? In
reality, the act of walking is quite intricate. We have all been made aware of this
recently from seeing television pictures of astronauts clumsily moving about in a
gravity-free chamber.

In normal gait, we use one leg to support ourselves and swing the other leg
forward. At the same time we let our body fall forward—actually lose our
balance. We are letting the force of gravity work here, but we smoothly control
this act of gravity by elongating the calf muscles of our supporting leg. When the
heel of the swinging leg strikes the floor, the lost balance is regained and the
weight of the body is quickly transferred onto the advanced leg. The continuous
forward motion of the body is, to a degree, a carry-over of a previously initiated
momentum (inertia). Thus, walking is a combination of economic use of the
forces of gravity and inertia, and of rapidly coordinated neuromuscular activity.

Another energy-saving determinant of gait is the double lock of the knee. A
young adult's knee bends during the swing phase (shortening the length of the

leg), but the knee straightens (is locked) the moment the heel strikes the floor. It bends a little immediately after the heelstrike, and straightens once again (the second lock) to support the superimposed weight of the body.

THE OLDER PERSON'S GAIT

The gait of a person of advanced age is different from that of a young adult. It is characterized by a more or less stooped trunk, a forward-craned neck and head, and a degree of flexion maintained in the hips and knees regardless of which leg is in the stance or swing phase. The steps are short.

Since the neuromuscular coordination of the older person is most impaired around the hips, he is not able to use to a full degree the determinants which could enable him to walk with less energy expenditure. His ability to lose and regain his physiological balance intermittently is markedly diminished, and for this reason he drags his feet along the floor during the swing phase (shuffling gait). The older person exploits the work of gravity very little. Instead, he has to use his own muscle power to walk. Also, the forward movement of the trunk is too slow and too hesitant to allow the work of inertia during forward propulsion.

When a young adult gets up from a low seat, he throws his trunk upward and forward, letting inertia correlate the movement of the trunk up and over the supporting feet which were in front of his trunk. An old person is not able to produce such a quick coordinated thrust. In order to stand up, he has to lean forward and put the center of gravity of his trunk exactly above the supporting surface of his feet before he lifts his body up; otherwise, he would fall backward.

The fact that most old people spend much of their time sitting, and that even their walking is done in a slightly knee- and hip-bent position, encourages the development of some degree of hip flexion contracture.

There is usually some deterioration of proprioceptive innervation in many persons of advanced age. They can augment the inadequate information about their relationship to the floor with the additional information they get via the cane and their hands. Experience has shown that these persons do better with heavier wooden canes or crutches than with lightweight aluminum ones, because the amount of sensory information they receive through their upper extremities is related to the weight of the cane or crutch and to the thickness of the handle.

IMPLICATIONS

What practical suggestions can we draw from the above considerations? Any person, particularly an older person, who has been bedfast for some time and who requires gait retraining must be gradually assisted to achieve the level where he can automatically judge correctly whether he is upright or not. This is accomplished by supervised or assisted standing-up exercises and ambulation. Sometimes it can be attained with power-building exercises for selected muscle groups.

Experience has shown that the most common factors which may cause an old person to lose his balance are: scatter rugs, slippery floors, and doorsills; hyperextension of the neck; sitting up, standing up, or turning quickly; and poor illumination at night. Scatter rugs, slippery floors, and doorsills are unstable surfaces of support on which old people are apt to lose control. And because of the slowing down of their neuromuscular reflexes they cannot regain their balance quickly. The older person is especially inclined to lose equilibrium while hyperextending his neck. For this reason, objects of daily need at home should not be placed on high shelves. Older people should be taught to sit up and to stand up slowly, and to wait a moment before proceeding to the next movement. Sudden turning around on the heel should be avoided by all means. Instead, old people should be taught to walk in a small circle to make a turn.

Visual information, even with impaired vision, is still the best guide old people have for reflexly ascertaining whether they are upright. Therefore, their houses should be well lighted, especially corridors and bathroom since older persons frequently get up at night to go to the bathroom. Leaning on a heavy object, such as a chair, a heavy cane, crutch, or walker may supply additional sensory information. There is no reason to overdo rehabilitation and train someone to get along without these ambulatory aids when they can supply such sensory assistance. Quick movement on one side of the visual field, as well as sudden, uneven illumination of the visual field of aged persons, may produce momentary abnormalities in their judgment of what is upright. For this reason, an old person with poor balance should stop and wait until someone who is in a hurry has passed him. Or, he should slow down when he has to go through doorways from a less illuminated corridor to a room brilliantly illuminated or one having daylight coming in a window.

All these precautions should be especially stressed if the person has a history of brain damage such as a cerebral vascular accident, Parkinson's disease, or a history of a fall resulting in a fractured hip. A special case in point is the elderly amputee. He can be at a marked disadvantage because of additional loss of proprioceptive data from the removed extremity, and because of his more limited locomotor control. Only about 10 percent of those over the age of 65 who have above-knee amputations learn to use an artificial limb successfully. On the other hand, more than 50 percent in this age group who have below-knee amputations learn to use an artificial limb. The above-knee amputee should be subjected to the following functional test to ascertain whether his remaining neuromuscular and cardiovascular abilities are good enough to enable him to benefit from an artificial limb: after three to four weeks of intensive crutch training, he must be able to walk with a good swingthrough gait and to climb stairs with the crutches without assistance. If he cannot do these, he is not able to use an artificial limb effectively.

The more we learn and understand about the locomotor abilities and limitations of both the healthy and the disabled aged, the more helpful we will be in giving them realistic advice and guidance. Nurses who work with older persons at home, in nursing homes, hospitals, or other care facilities know how serious the consequences of falls may be. They can do much to help persons of advanced age to accept and adapt to changing physical limitations, and to develop habits that will insure easier and safer walking.

What do size and resiliency of muscles and muscle tone have to do with ambulation?

How much thinking do you do as you take each step?

How does the posture differ for the four age groups previously mentioned?

Define proprioception and state how this relates to walking.

Talk with persons who have had falls: children, adults, and old people. What caused the fall? What injuries resulted? What can be or has been done to prevent a similar incident?

Why is a walker more helpful to an elderly person than to a younger person requiring assistance with ambulation?

21.
Stimulation Through Remotivation

Glee Gamble Lyon

*What is the purpose of a remotivation group? How would you feel
about discussing clouds or windmills with adults but at a child's
level of understanding?*

In many hospitals there are patients who spend their days sitting, pacing, or just
lying on their beds. Their day-to-day lives are filled with feelings of isolation,
apathy, lethargy, loneliness, and even uselessness and hopelessness. Those who
work with these patients often find themselves feeling useless or hopeless, too.
However, many of these patients can be reached through the use of remotivation
techniques.

A remotivation group can stimulate a person's interest in his environment,
increase his communication skills, and help him learn or relearn a wide variety of
skills.

EXPECTATION

The whole atmosphere surrounding a remotivation group should be positive: this
is an hour that not only is "safe," it also will be fun! Something different is
going to happen. This is the attitude the group leaders must convey to patients
whose days are generally filled with apathy and indifference.

The feeling of expectation can be enhanced by the setting in which the group
meets. Certainly, the room should be comfortable, with windows and plenty of
light. Chairs arranged in a circle, or, even better, in a horseshoe shape, make it

128

possible for the leader to stand toward one end of the group without having her back to any one member, yet move easily from one member to another in the group. This arrangement will also increase interaction among group members.

If possible, a room or building different from the place where members spend most of their days should be used.

METHOD

The structure or method used depends on the patient's level of functioning and the purpose of the group. If remotivation groups are new to leader and members, both will be helped to make this experience more successful if group meetings follow a very defined structure, such as that developed by Dorothy Hoskins Smith. In this approach, each meeting with the group focuses on an objective topic and follows five basic steps.

1. CLIMATE OF ACCEPTANCE The group begins, after all members are seated, with the group leader introducing herself and then going around the group and greeting each patient individually. The group leader moves close to each person, establishes eye contact, and either shakes hands or touches each patient's arm if this is tolerated. She then says each patient's name, and gives him a greeting, such as "Hello, Mike, I'm glad you could come," or "Helen, you look very nice today," or "Thank you, Ron, for carrying my box to the meeting." The comments and individual recognition convey to each member that *he* is wanted in this group.

2. A BRIDGE TO THE REAL WORLD After the greeting, to further establish a positive climate, and give the meeting structure, the leader tells the group members what they will be doing today. After members are accustomed to remotivation and feel they can trust the leader, they can begin to enjoy an element of surprise but, initially, they need to know what to expect from the time they will spend together. The leader can say, "Today we are going to discover how a windmill works." Or, she can ask several simple questions that lead patients to discover what the topic is.

Group Leader: Today, as we walked to the group, did anyone look up at the sky? What did you see?

Members: The sun.

Group Leader: Yes! And did anyone see something else?

Members: Clouds.

Group Leader: Good, today we are going to talk about clouds.

A poem is often read at this time because many patients respond to rhythm and rhyme, and also because poems present word pictures. The poem needs to be about the topic, fairly short, and easily understood. Books of children's poems are an excellent source. After the group leader or several group members have read poems, the leader can ask a few questions about the poems which will help introduce the topic.

3. THE WORLD IN WHICH WE LIVE The main part of the meeting is devoted to exploring a topic together. The leader does not give information to group members; rather she helps them share information they already have or, together, discover new information. Although the leader's main purpose is not to lecture or give information, it is important that she be both interested in the topic chosen and know something about it.

Almost any topic can be used. Most can be presented in very elementary fashion for patients whose attention span is short or whose intelligence or education is limited or geared to stimulate patients with alert minds and more education.

The topic should be specific. The subject "animals" is too broad and too hard to organize around a few main points. However, if in one session the topic is "cats," all members at the end of the session should be better acquainted with this animal.

4. WORK OF WORLD After a topic has been explored, conversation can be directed toward the type of work or jobs that are related to the topic. This step helps a patient think about work in relation to himself, or gives him an opportunity to share past experiences with others.

5. CLIMATE OF APPRECIATION To end a meeting, the group leader and members summarize what has been discussed. The leader then thanks each person for coming and tells when they will meet again. The session can also end with cookies and punch or coffee and a social period. Often, after the structured meeting, while drinking punch, several patients might start a conversation among themselves about the topic or about something unrelated, or the leader might help them further explore one aspect of the day's topic, trying to include several patients in very informal discussion.

HANDLING BEHAVIORS

A leader will need to feel reasonably comfortable and sure of herself before she can help other group members feel comfortable and enjoy the session. In a group of non-participating patients it is easy for the leader who gets no response to fill the silence. If she is not careful she sets up a pattern of both asking and answering her own questions.

Keeping to a well outlined plan will help to reduce a leader's anxiety and a few well-stated key questions written on small note cards will help the leader who finds herself stumped as to what to do next.

Visual aids are an effective anxiety-reducer because they focus group members' attention away from the leader to a physical object. In addition, it is easier for members to respond on a physical level—looking, touching, smelling.

An excellent device to help leader and group members forget their anxieties is a live animal—a cat, dog, guinea pig, or parrot in a cage. However, other objects—shoes, hats, leaves, even pictures—also will help to reduce anxiety and stimulate group discussion.

Many nonverbal patients get a great deal out of a group by just listening, seeing, feeling, and exploring objects. The leader can direct questions to the nonverbal member occasionally so that he knows she is interested in him, but if the member still feels unable to contribute, the leader can decrease his anxiety by saying, "Maybe you can tell us later" or "Maybe you'll have something to say later." This lets the person know there is no pressure to talk now and plants the expectation that at some later time he will take a more active part.

At times one patient tends to monopolize group discussion. The leader can support this person but also limit his contributions by saying, "Thank you, Connie, you gave us one good answer. Who knows another reason why we. . .?"

The patient who has an idea but has difficulty in expressing it may ramble, wandering far from the topic. He needs special help. The leader can usually let this member continue until she has an idea of what he means. Then the leader can validate her understanding of the comments while stating for the group: "Do you mean that one important difference between. . . ." Or she can summarize in a few simple statements, "Mr. S. just said that. . . ." This usually supports the person and, at the same time, prevents other group members from becoming confused and losing interest.

If a member tries to use the meeting time to relate such concerns as "Nurse, I'm going home today" or "I think I'm taking too much medicine, will the doctor be on the ward today," the leader can recognize the concern but also limit its discussion, by saying, "We need to talk about that after the group meeting; right now we are talking about clocks." The leader then, of course, must be sure to find the time to help the individual talk about his own concerns later.

The same approach is used for a patient who becomes delusional: "This is China and I'm the Princess of Hong Kong; everyone is to go before the King." The leader can say rather firmly, "Joyce, we are talking about clocks right now." If the member is still unable to participate or at least remain quiet long enough to allow the rest of the group to participate, the leader might say, "Joyce, the group is talking about clocks; you're talking about something else and it is disturbing the rest of us. Either be quiet or you will have to leave." A patient who becomes too disruptive should be removed from the group so that other members can continue their meeting.

Members who function at quite different levels can both contribute to and learn from the same group. The leader might direct a very concrete question to one group member, "What color is this soldier's uniform?" To the rest of the group, the leader might ask, "Why is the soldier's uniform a green-brown color?" The first member's answer thus serves as the basis for others to build upon.

Members whose life experiences vary widely also can contribute to the same group. One member might describe the seaside from a picture even though he has never been there. Another, who has been to the seaside, can share what he did there from firsthand experience.

VARIATIONS

Basic remotivation techniques can be used for different purposes or on different levels. For example, on a men's ward, eight patients with very poor personal appearance were formed into a group to talk about grooming.

Remotivation groups for patients can be organized around the accomplishment of a task. On one ward, many women patients, although capable of functioning at a higher level at home than in the hospital, tended to spend most of their time lying on their beds. Attempts to involve them in occupational therapy projects had been unsuccessful. Ten of these women were formed into a group and told to plan, prepare, and give a bingo party for the rest of the women on the ward.

Such short-term groups do create little islands of active participation and serve the purpose of stimulating and involving patients for the length of the meeting; however, to reach a higher goal of actually changing attitudes and behavior, remotivation groups must be continuing.

At the very least, a remotivation group interrupts the monotony of a seemingly endless day, provides reality contact, and something fun to do. The potential of a remotivation group seemingly could reach as high as the limits of the leader's imagination and creativity and group members' potential for growth.

The leader of a remotivation group probably faces many moments of anxiety and discomfort in attempting to get group members to respond. Gather a group together and try some of these methods. Reread the last paragraph. Keep your goals simple at first but do make the effort.

Describe two clinical settings where you feel patients could use this type of group work. Who could conduct the groups in each setting?

PART III

COPING WITH CRISES

Nurses have come a long way in incorporating psychiatric nursing skills into their everyday patient care because they recognize how each person is beset with emotional problems and how these problems affect their physical well being. They also know how to predict the course that an emotional shock (such as death of a loved one) will take and how to be helpful along the way. Patient behavior is now viewed objectively instead of merely endured or resisted. A minor loss — or what seems minor to a nurse — can be a major crisis event to the patient because of whatever previous experiences it summons to his conscious mind.

A crisis event occurs when a person suffers a loss — whether it be of a loved one, a part of his body, or of his role in life. The reaction that results is referred to as the *grief reaction* because the person grieves over the loss. This is a very abbreviated definition but one that you may find helpful if these phrases are new to you. The articles in this group all deal with crises events and the grief reaction.

THE PROCESS

22.

Grief and Depression

Otto F. Thaler

Dr. Thaler views grief as a normal and necessary phase of living. In his article he makes frequent reference to Dr. Engel's work on grief. Dr. Engel's article can be found in the September 1964 issue of the American Journal of Nursing. The behaviors that nurses need to anticipate and recognize are clearly described by Dr. Thaler, however. You will probably wish to refer back to this article frequently as you care for grieving patients and help them avoid depressions.

Hence, loathed Melancholy,
Of Cerberus and blackest Midnight born,
In Stygian cave forlorn,
'Mongst horrid shapes, and shrieks,
and sights unholy.

John Milton: L'Allegro, 1632

Grief fills the room up of my absent child,
Lies in his bed, walks up and down with me,
Puts on his pretty looks, repeats his words,
Remembers me of all his gracious parts,
Stuffs out his vacant garments with his form;
Then have I reason to be fond of grief.

William Shakespeare: King John, 1596

These two quotations − one from Shakespeare, the other from Milton − epitomize the difference between the two related, ubiquitous human experiences of grief and depression. The subject is as old as man's capacity for self-observation, as old as man's ability to record and puzzle over his inner experiences and those of his fellowman.

The prominent similar feature of grief and depression is a disturbance in mood. Man's preoccupation with this most painful of his moods is attested to by the following list of terms to describe it: Depression, grief, sadness, despair, blues, helplessness, feeling low, gloom, despondency, mourning, cheerlessness, listlessness, hopelessness, dejection, heartsickness, sorrow, anguish, joylessness, unhappiness, melancholy, woe, oppression.

The ancient Greeks knew of grief as did those who lived in Biblical times. Both also knew of its relative − loathed melancholy, or depression − as something different, something irrational and therefore frightening.

The Greeks tried to grapple with this puzzle in their mythology. There they tried to explain this awesome and terrifying exacerbation of the common mood of sadness. In its agonizing starkness the dark madness could only be dealt with through projection − through attributing its genesis to external, supernatural, divine influences. At the same time the wisdom of the mythmaker saw clearly and compassionately into the heart of the sufferer.

One tale, the story of Queen Niobe, attempts to account for the inscrutable ways of fate and man's terrifying reaction to it. Queen Niobe had seven sons and seven daughters, of whom she was inordinately proud. She derided the goddess Leto for having only two children, Apollo and Artemis. In revenge for the arrogance of the mortal queen, Leto's two children killed all of Niobe's fourteen. Niobe's sorrow was so extreme that she turned into a statue, frozen forever in the attitude of grief. Her only signs of life were the tears which streamed down the statue's face.

Here is the dawning perception of a difference between grief and depression in terms of their relative duration and the degree of incapacitation associated with each. Here is awareness, too, of an etiological role which aggression plays in the genesis of many depressions and of how aggression is turned against the self by guilt and an eternally punishing harsh conscience. For our purpose, the most important insight offered by this story is the recognition of loss as the central precipitating factor in depression. Niobe's diagnosis: a case of depressive stupor.

The Bible gives us King Saul, who, rejected by the Lord and plagued by guilt, became psychotically depressed. David, in the first recorded instance of music therapy, is said to have cured him by playing the harp. Like so many other uncontrolled therapeutic experiments, the miraculous treatment seems to have coincided with a spontaneous remission. Saul experienced further losses in his life; he became seriously depressed and finally died by his own hand. Thus the Bible teaches us that a psychotic depression is self-limited and that it is liable to recur.

Many of the great of the world suffered from recurrent depressive episodes. Abraham Lincoln, following the death of Ann Rutledge, experienced a serious suicidal depression, from which he slowly recovered in the care of friends. In contrast to Saul's music therapy, his treatment was occupational therapy: "cornhusking, cutting wood, picking apples, digging potatoes, doing light chores around the house." He had other, less severe depressive episodes throughout his life.

How do we view these matters today? What similarities do we see between grief and depression? How do we attempt to distinguish between them? And why do we find it clinically necessary to make such a distinction?

The definitions which I shall offer you reflect a frame of reference which is shared by many clinicians, but not by all. As in the case of Tweedledum and Tweedledee in *Alice in Wonderland,* the words "grief" and "depression" mean what the physician evaluating and treating the patient choose them to mean for the purpose of making a clinical differentiation and ordering observable phenomena so that he can deal with them clinically. [I hope this statement will help us to avoid arguing or worrying about words and will, instead, enable us to focus on the clinical material.]

The major factor which grief and depression have in common is that at the psychological level they both represent a reaction to loss. They also share certain phenomenological features at certain stages of their natural history. The ideational content may also be similar at certain stages of the development of these two conditions. Beyond these points of likeness, however, they differ significantly. They should, since we consider the one "normal" and the other "pathological."

In the discussion of "normal" grief I shall draw on the work of Engel, Schmale, and Greene of our Department and on a discussion of this work recently prepared by Axelrod.

Grief is a response to loss. It is best known to all of us as a response to the loss through death or separation of a loved person, but it occurs following the loss of anything, tangible or intangible, which is highly valued. This may be a material possession, a position of status, a prized faculty, or a place one is forced to leave. Thus, homesickness is a most common form of grief.

The ability to experience grief at any such loss is gradually formed in the course of normal development. The acquisition of the capacity for grieving is closely related to the acquisition of the capacity for developing meaningful object relationships. It is, we might say, its reverse aspect. ("It is better to have loved and lost than never to have loved at all.") Thus, those who are able to form relationships at all become attached even to situations and places which are less than optimal and grieve for them, albeit briefly, even when moving on to better conditions.

For a number of years my family and I lived in a very small and eventually very crowded little house. We finally were able to move from there into a comparatively capacious and luxurious new home. The children were thrilled and excited. "When will we move? I can't wait." The great day came. We moved, and each child was installed in his very own room. When it came time to tuck the children in on that first night in the new house, all three of them were sitting up in bed and crying, "I wish we were back in the old house. I miss it so."

Normal, "successful" grieving, according to Engel, has three phases, which are especially evident in the case of grief following the death of a loved one. The first is characterized by the terms *shock and disbelief.* The almost universal exclamation upon hearing of a sudden loss is "Oh no!" How many of us recall saying just that on November 22, 1963, when first hearing of President Kennedy's death.

Each individual has his own idiosyncratic style of denial of an unbearable reality. Cultural factors play a part in determining how dramatically or how subtly this denial is expressed. For example, some persons, who seem to be able to accept stoically what has happened, continue to function and may even attempt to comfort others, less close to the deceased, in their grief. Louis Auchincloss describes most sensitively such a person in his recent novel *The Rector of Justin.* The setting of the book is a boys' school. The narrator, a young master who has recently come to the school, is befriended by the headmaster's dying wife. When she finally dies, the young man is grief-stricken. When he goes to the headmaster, Dr. Prescott, to offer his condolences, he tells him of the last words he heard the dying woman speak. The headmaster's reaction is recorded as follows:

Without smiling, he winked at me. "How like Harriet. How
gloriously like her. To go out on such a note of protest. Thank
you for telling me that." He rose and reached his hand across the
desk to me. I grasped it and then to my horror I began to sob. I
covered my face and sobbed.
"It's all right, dear boy," I heard him say in the kindest of tones.
"You loved my wife, and I deeply appreciate it."
Dr. Prescott came around to my side of the desk and put a hand on
my shoulder. "It's a good thing to have feeling, Brian. One can't
really control it unless one has it, can one? You'll be all right. You
have a great deal to give to others, and I think your calling may be
a true one. But I don't think you're ready yet. I think maybe a year
or two at Justine may be precisely what you need."
I rubbed my eyes, grasped his hand again and hurried from the
room. I, who should have been consoling, had asked consolation
and had received it munificently!

Engel summarizes this phase:

Distinctive of this initial phase are the attempts to protect oneself
against the effects of the overwhelming stress by raising the
threshold against its recognition or against the painful feeling
evoked thereby.

The second phase of grief is characterized by *developing awareness*. Its onset
may be very soon after the bereavement, or it may take considerable time to
develop. In this phase reality inexorably begins to assert itself. Awareness of the
pain of the loss becomes acute and with it comes awareness of the terrible
emptiness which the loss has caused. There may be anger toward others who
have been close to the dead person. Self-injury or self-destructive behavior may
occur here. Both the anger toward others and that expressed toward the self
through self-injury or gestures of self-destruction are displacements of anger
belonging to the dead person for his desertion. The anguish and the feeling of
having been injured by the beloved dead are most movingly expressed in the last
song of Robert Schumann's song cycle *Women's Love and Suffering*. The cycle
describes, in several songs, the nodal points in the life of a very happily married
woman – courtship, marriage, the birth of a son. The last song describes the
woman's feelings after her beloved husband dies. She says "Now, for the first
time, you have grievously hurt me. You sleep, you hard, you cruel man. You
sleep the sleep of death. The world is empty."

Finally, but importantly, in this stage there is crying. There should be crying.
Grief without tears is incomplete. Tearless grief indicates that the work of
mourning has not been finished. It may indicate excessively ambivalent feelings
toward the deceased and undue guilt on the part of the mourner. Pathology may
eventuate, such as severe depression, which may ensue gradually or may appear
for the first time on the anniversary of the death. The need for the expression of
grief either openly or in private has also long been recognized by poets. "Give
sorrow words: the grief that does not speak whispers the o'er-fraught heart and
bids it break." (Shakespeare: Macbeth, 1605.)

The third phase of grief is that of *restitution*. This completes the work of
mourning. Engel says:

The institutionalization of the mourning experience in terms of the
various rituals of a funeral help to initiate the recovery processes.
First it involves a gathering together of family and friends who
mutually share the loss although not all to the same degree. At the
same time there is acknowledgement of the need for support of the
most stricken survivors whose regression is accepted. In this setting,

an overt or conscious expression of aggression is reduced to a minimum. Many of the rituals of the funeral serve the important function
of emphasizing clearly and unequivocally the reality of the death, the
denial of which cannot be allowed to go on if recovery from the loss
is to take place . . . . In addition, individual religious and spiritual
beliefs offer recourse in various ways to the support of a more
powerful beneficent figure or provide the basis for the expectation
of some kind of reunion after death and the expiation of guilt.

Here again we can refer to a mourning experience which we all shared. "The
institutionalization of the mourning experience" — how many of us sat through
the three or four days of President Kennedy's funeral rites, and how many of us
felt relieved and purged at the end of this period! We cried and we mourned
when they played "Hail to the Chief," when we watched Mrs. Kennedy and the
children in their superbly controlled grief, and when we saw little John salute his
father for the last time.

Another feature of this period of restitution is the elevation of the memory
of the dead person to a degree of perfection, devoid of negative features, which
overlooks some of the realities of his actual personality. It takes many months
for the mourner to be able to take a more realistic view of the deceased — it may
never be accomplished altogether. Remember the spate of adulatory, hero-
worshiping books and mementos which appeared shortly after President
Kennedy's death and which has continued to the present? However, as time
passes there also seems to be an increasing tendency to try and see the man with
all his faults behind the myth produced by the work of mourning of a whole
nation. Thus, gradually new objects take the place of the lost one, and often
within a year mourning is completed.

Now — *depression.* To illustrate the discussion of the problem of grief I have
used examples from literature and the arts and from commonly shared historical
experience, because grief is a common, normal, and necessary experience of all
men everywhere. To illustrate depression I shall use clinical examples, thus
emphasizing the fact that although it is extremely common, it is a pathological
elaboration of grief — related to but by no means the same as grief.

Depression, like grief, is a reaction to loss. However, whereas grief is almost
always the response to a real loss, depression is the response to a loss which is
basically rooted in fantasy, which is symbolic, threatened, or imagined. The loss
may appear to be a realistic one, but as the reaction to it continues beyond that
of normal grief in duration as well as intensity, closer investigation will point to
factors other than the realistic one of, let us say, the loss of a loved person —
factors which feed and perpetuate the depression.

A clinical example will illustrate this point. The patient was an elderly
woman, severely and profoundly depressed, with all of the classical signs —
anorexia, insomnia, motor retardation, weight loss, and a deepgoing mood

change to hopelessness, worthlessness, and helplessness. Her favorite daughter had married a British subject, and now, a year later, the couple was to leave for England. In this setting the mother's depression broke out. The only thing the daughter thought she could do was to call off the move to England. Her husband obtained a job in the United States. They brought the glad tidings to mother. There was no change whatever in the mother's depression.

This woman's initial response to the imminent separation from her daughter was already "too much" — so often a sign to the clinician that psychopathology is present. She reacted, not like an adult in response to an inevitable separation (which should have had some elements of joy for her, in terms of her daughter's successful achievement of adult status), but more as if she herself were still a child being separated prematurely from her mother. And furthermore — the clincher, so to speak, in our diagnostic evaluation — the reality of the daughter's remaining in this country had no influence on the effect which the fancied, fantasied separation had had on the patient's mood and behavior.

The kind of loss to which the patient reacts with depression is often much less apparent, much more in the category of a loss which is meaningful only to the individual patient in terms of his own idiosyncratic life experience. One man's loss may be meaningless, unintelligible to another man. I would like to emphasize the importance for clinical personnel in any specialty field to become skillful in detecting and understanding the more subtle kinds of depression, which are often masked or obscured by other primary, somatic conditions. This relationship may be illustrated by the case histories of two patients, Mr. B and Mr. D.

Mr. B was admitted to one of the psychiatric wards at Strong Memorial Hospital following one of the most dramatic suicide attempts I have ever heard of. He was a stocky, red-faced, rugged-looking man in his middle forties. On the day of his admission he had driven his car out to the airport, parked it next to one of the hangars, and taken off in his own little two-seater plane. He flew around a little, then turned back and deliberately dove his plane at his car with the intent of destroying plane, car, and himself. He succeeded in his first two objectives and, in addition, damaged the hangar. He himself walked away from the crash. The other patient, Mr. D, was an old man in his early eighties who was admitted to my floor as a surgical boarder.

He, too, had made a suicidal attempt that day — one that was less dramatic than Mr. B's, but no less serious and more nearly successful. He had taken his straight razor and deeply slashed his throat from ear to ear, cutting through the trachea but somehow miraculously missing the great vessels.

What did these two have in common, the rugged amateur-pilot and the octogenarian? Here are their stories as they emerged during their hospitalization.

First, Mr. B: In retrospect both the patient and his family had noticed the onset of despondency a few weeks back when it first became evident that his very painful shoulder — painful to the point of immobility — was not yielding to treatment. It had finally been put in a cast. Mr. B therefore had not worked in several weeks. Mr. B operated, in his own words, the "largest Goddam steam-shovel in New York" — a job which he obviously gloried in. He had hurt his shoulder when lifting an oildrum.

He was later said to have had a capsulitis, which takes eight weeks to subside regardless of what treatment is used. He did not know this, and when his arm was no better after four weeks of various treatments he had begun to believe that he would never be able to use that arm again — certainly not to drive the biggest steam-shovel in New York. Mr. B was a compulsive "he" man. He was a hunter, a fisherman, a rugged outdoors type. He owned a speedboat, a fast car, a little plane. His whole life was dedicated to the reiterated demonstration of his masculinity through the pursuit of these virile activities, of which his work was merely the most outstanding one. The imagined threat of the future loss of these capacities produced the profound depression which went unrecognized and which eventuated in his act of desperation.

Mr. D also had a medical problem. Two or three months prior to admission he had had a cerebrovascular accident resulting in paralysis of his right side, from which he was recovering only very gradually. Mr. D had never been sick a day in his life until then; he had not missed a day's work in fifty years. He was one of the last remaining blacksmiths in Rochester and had worked till the day of his stroke at a local industrial concern, where he kept all kinds of wheel-bearing equipment in working condition. Mr. D was a widower who supported himself and lived by himself until his illness forced him to move in with a daughter, who gladly took care of him. He had been assured that he would at least regain his capacity to navigate, but progress was slow and he, the man of independence, was increasingly distraught at having to have someone else attend to even his most intimate bodily needs. His increasing despondency was read as crankiness. In a setting in which he had fallen while trying to reach the toilet by himself, had had to be helped up, had been scolded and then toileted by his daughter, he reached for the razor and almost put an end to a life he considered worthless.

What do these two cases have in common? They both teach us that the loss of function, the loss of self-esteem, the loss of a cherished self-image may have as disastrous results as the loss of a loved one or the loss of property. These two cases teach us to look for those factors in our patients' lives which are meaningful for *them* and essential for them and then to direct our therapeutic and management efforts accordingly. Neither Mr. B nor Mr. D needed any treatment except supportive psychotherapeutic measures to help them in their recovery. Mr. B was clearly instructed as to the self-limited nature of his condition and given careful and detailed explanations regarding the treatment of his injured shoulder. The shoulder got better as predicted, and Mr. B shortly thereafter was able to leave the hospital. Mr. D, after his wound healed, was started on intensive physiotherapy and soon was pushing his walker around the floor for as long each day as we would allow it — determined to get on his feet and make his way to the bathroom. He, too, did well in follow-up.

Grief, then, is a universal, normal, developmentally-evolved adaptive process. Its progress in three predictable phases is essential to enable the individual to deal adaptively with the disturbance of the psychological equilibrium inevitably caused by object loss. Grief is self-limited, gradually diminishing over the period of a year. Except in its very early, acute phase it is not incapacitating, and even in the early phase it may not grossly interfere with the individual's normal functioning in many areas of his life.

Depression represents a malfunction of this normal mechanism of adaptation to object loss. While the loss may be apparent and understandable to the observer, it has to the patient special meaning in fantasy, or symbolically with reference to the past. This meaning is not available to the observer and the patient is unaware of it. It is this special meaning, unrelated to the reality of the loss (regardless of its apparent severity) which triggers the special reaction, depression. This is a catastrophic response to what, in the patient's frame of reference is a catastrophic loss, regardless of what it seems like to the observer, who may regard it as trivial or not apparent at all. Depression, which except in its grossest psychotic form may initially resemble grief, does not enter the phase of restitution within a few weeks or days of its onset. It is prolonged, it is severe, and it is increasingly incapacitating in all areas of the patient's life.

Those who work with patients must recognize normal grief when they see it and not interfere with its normal course. They must also be alert to the signs of depression, so that measures can be taken to guard against the dangers of depression and treatment can be instituted as soon as possible after it has been diagnosed.

How does grief differ from depression? List in two columns some signs and symptoms of each.

What signs and symptoms would you expect a nurse to notice as signs of depression for Mr. D and Mr. B.? What actions would you take? How would you implement a patient-care conference for these patients? How would you go about evaluating the effect of your actions?

Compare the actions you listed here with those suggested in the next selection by Dr. Ujhely.

23.
Grief and Depression

Gertrud B. Ujhely

*In the following article you will learn more about behavior as Dr.
Ujhely clearly describes nursing actions to take when working with
patients experiencing a loss, those who are depressed, and those
with long-term illnesses. She makes frequent reference to Dr.
Gerald Caplan's book* Principles of Preventive Psychiatry, *New
York, Basic Books, 1964.*

Grief and depression are conditions which bring into sharp focus the special
contribution of nursing, namely, sustaining the patient in his subjective
experience so that he may be able to cope with it, integrate it into his past
experience, and, it is to be hoped, learn from it and grow through it. It is also
possible that in some cases of depression (although probably not in all) the
nurse, aided by the information in Dr. Thaler's article, can distinguish this
pathological phenomenon from normal grief and thus be instrumental in the
initiation of early treatment for it.

In any event, the nurse can be aware of the depressive components in any
grief and the loss components in most instances of depression. Then, by means
of nursing interventions directed toward helping a person to become aware of
and experience his grief, she may be able to forestall the development of
depression. She may also be able to protect the depressed person from utilizing
disastrous exits to escape from his intolerable state. Finally, she may perhaps be
able to help a person to move through the various stages of grief and reach a
state in which he can make use of the rehabilitative service available to him.

These opportunities for nursing to make its specific contribution to those

*From "Grief and Depression" by Gertrud B. Ujhely, published in Volume V, No.
2 of* Nursing Forum. *Copyright © 1966 by Nursing Publications, Inc.
Reproduced, with permission, from* Nursing Forum.

who are afflicted with grief or depression can be discussed in light of the three modes of prevention which are used in the public health approach to physical illness and lately, in the approach to emotional states also.

PRIMARY PREVENTION

How can nurses help to forestall or mitigate impending grief and, possibly, help to prevent the occurrence of depression? One way is to help a person with an impending loss to talk about the loss and what it means to him. This anticipatory guidance, as Gerald Caplan calls it, may desensitize the person somewhat to the massive impact of the loss. It may also, perhaps, give the person some perspective to his value system so that the loss, when it occurs, is not such a crucial one for him.

Take for instance a mother who sees her only role in life as being the person on whom her dependent children can lean; in other words, her purpose in life is to be needed. In a few months her youngest child, her "baby," will be going to school, and she will not be needed by her children in the same way as before. Unless she comes to grips with this fact, she is liable to go through a grief period; even worse, if she is unable to see herself in any light other than the accustomed one, she may go into a depression.

The public health nurse can help this mother by giving her an opportunity to talk about the impending drastic change in her life. True, the mother may not be able to accept this offer; even thinking about the future may be too threatening for her. The nurse must respect this reluctance, but she can leave an opening for such a talk by letting the mother know that should she wish to discuss the subject in the future the nurse will be available to her.

If, however, the mother responds by telling about what, to her, is an impending loss of her child to the world, the nurse can help her by accepting the fact that she feels the way she does, even though her point of view may seem rather narrow, perhaps even selfish. The nurse should acknowledge that this change will be a real one and that it is desirable to think about it beforehand. At the same time, it may be possible to throw a little doubt on the bulwark of the mother's value system — not enough to topple it over, but enough so that she will need to look for new props which will enable her to sustain the threat of the oncoming event. The nurse might ask her to think about whether the way her child needs her now is the only way one can be needed, or whether there are other ways, such as being home when the child comes from school, listening to what he has to say about his experiences in school, being available to help him with his homework, helping him to look the way he wants to look in front of his peers, and so on.

The nurse might also very carefully suggest to this mother that she take a look at herself. Undoubtedly, one of her great virtues is to meet the needs of her children, but surely she must have other virtues; she has not always been a mother. Perhaps the time has come for her to take stock of these other virtues which, owing to her childrens' demands and needs, have been lying dormant for so long.

Of course, all that the nurse can do is sow these seeds. To see to it that they fall on soil which can imbed them and help them to sprout is beyond her jurisdiction and power. Moreover, the nurse must watch herself so that her own need to help does not become a weapon instead of a seed, so that she does not engage in a power struggle with this mother and attempt to force her to believe what she, the nurse, thinks is right. Such a struggle would divert the mother's energies from trying to cope with her impending loss experience to a defense against the onslaught of the nurse's advice.

Variations on this theme of impending loss are the parents whose children are about to get married and the man or woman who is about to retire. The latter situation might have particular implications for the nurse working in industry.

Both the public health nurse and the hospital nurse have many opportunities to give anticipatory guidance to relatives of patients who are about to die. In such a situation, the nurse may be able to prepare the family for what is likely to happen. She can ask them whether they have ever witnessed a death before. She can give them an opportunity to talk about it and to ask questions.

The nurse should not be surprised, however, if the relative of a dying patient seems to ignore completely his present situation and starts telling her about a past loss. Each emotional experience a person has resounds in the recesses of repressed, past similar experiences; therefore, any impending loss revives all unfinished business concerning previous losses. Moreover, since our culture makes it very difficult for us to live through the various stages of the grief process successfully and in full measure, the chances are that most people have a large reservoir of unfinished business relating to former losses. In the case of a dying patient's relative, the nurse may be the first person to whom he can talk about his unfinished grief-work. By helping him to abreact his past grief, she may make it possible for him to deal, when the time comes, with the situation at hand instead of having to protect himself from experiencing it because of the fear of an onslaught of reawakened memories. Thus the nurse may be able to protect him from a depression, even though she cannot magically remove his just cause for grief.

There is another way in which we as nurses can, perhaps, forestall depression in relatives of patients who are bound to die, for example, the parents of a child with leukemia or a wife or husband whose spouse is in the last stages of a fatal disease. Often these people seem devoid of affect. They talk about the impending death of their loved one in a matter-of-fact way and seem to go about their daily affairs as if nothing were happening to them. The nurse may think that they are heartless, or she may want to help them by encouraging them to express emotion — "It is all right to cry." The fact is that these relatives need support for their present lack of emotion, or rather for the dissociation they are experiencing between emotion and mind and action. Often they conceive of themselves as monsters, as heartless beings, devoid of love for someone so very close to them. The nurse can support them in this apparent coldness by explaining to them that this is a protection nature has provided so that they *can* go about their business, *can* keep their household together and not, by their despair, cause double abandonment of those members of the household who will survive. By encouraging them at this time to produce emotion the nurse could counteract the protective mechanism which helps them and their loved ones to survive the terrific onslaught which lies in store for them.

Again, the nurse in the hospital is often on hand to prevent serious depression in patients who are about to undergo a surgical intervention that is likely to make them feel unworthy of themselves in light of their value system. Examples might be patients who are about to have a breast biopsy which may mean a radical mastectomy or merely the excision of a cyst and patients with impending hysterectomies, prostatectomies, or amputations. By implicit convention these patients are often expected to keep a stiff upper lip, to undergo these self-threatening procedures with a minimum of fuss because they are the rational measures to take. Also, many of these patients react to the assault upon their self-system with a delayed serious depression or sometimes even with a full-blown paranoid reaction.

The nurse should make herself available to such a patient in case he wants to talk about the meaning the surgical procedure has for him. In other words, she should be alert to clues that the patient wants to talk with her or she might create an opening by asking him if there is anything he would like to ask about or talk about. Of course, as in all other instances, it is the patient's privilege to accept or ignore this offer. Whether the nurse is successful in these talks depends not only on her skill, but also on the time she has available for discussion and the degree to which the patient's stiff-upper-lip attitude is ingrained in him.

SECONDARY PREVENTION

For the nurse to engage in secondary prevention which is directed toward reducing the duration of the condition, implies that she is instrumental in early diagnosis, referral, and treatment of the condition. It means that whenever she has a hunch that a patient's grief-reaction is more than just grief, is somewhat inappropriate, is more tinged with resentment, or is marked by a greater degree of retardation in physical and thought processes than is to be expected, she should report this hunch to the responsible family member, to the doctor who is treating the patient, and to the nurse in charge of the unit or the service. Also, by listening to her own hunches the nurse may often forestall disastrous escapes from an unrecognized state of depression.

How can the nurse who is taking care of a patient suffering from severe grief or an acute depression help him to endure his state, to use his limited available energies constructively so that he does not unnecessarily prolong his agony? The nurse must be careful that she does not fall into the patient's own pitfall, that is, that she does not take the attitude that he should not feel the way he does, that he has so much to live for, that he is being unfair to himself and others. By accepting the patient's experiences, the nurse can perhaps help him to accept his despair — his "desperately wanting to be himself" or "desperately wanting to be anything but himself," but definitely *not* wanting to be in the actual state in which he finds himself. She can show him she understands that he feels hopeless, unworthy, guilty, but at the same time she should try to help him to see that these feelings are defenses, attempts to escape from his actual sensation of being utterly trapped. She can encourage him to give credence to the feeling of being trapped rather than to the conclusion that his situation must be a hopeless one. She can validate with him his feeling that others despise him, but she must also remind him that this feeling does not mean that others really do despise him. He may feel unworthy of being loved and therefore not perceive the love of others, but that does not mean the love does not exist.

Also, the nurse can encourage the patient not to make unnecessary, unreasonable demands on himself, such as pretending that he feels much better than he actually does feel, or expecting of himself that he should enjoy occupational therapy or recreational therapy activities at a time when all his energy and attention is taken up by his inner conflicts. Yet at the same time she must encourage him to go through the motions of those activities, even though they seem meaningless to him, for getting mobilized will in the long run help him to get out of the trap of his depression.

Taking care of depressed patients is not an easy task; the impossible demands they tend to make on life, on others, and on themselves are particularly irritating. They are like the prisoner who shakes the bars in front of his windows in impotent fury, completely unaware of the fact that the door behind him is unlocked, waiting for him to walk out, as it were. It is easy to get angry with a depressed patient or to resent him for the feeling of helplessness he creates in others, but if the nurse becomes angry or resentful, she defeats her own purpose and becomes servant to the patient's pathology.

Perhaps we nurses need to tell ourselves again and again that it is not our job to cure the patient; we can only offer him support in his prison cell. Unless we are psychotherapists as well as nurses, it is not up to us to scrutinize with the patient what has caused his depression. Rather, our task is to help him to tolerate his state, to live through it, so that he may be able to profit from the therapy, somatic or psychological, which is offered him. We can do this by validating for him again and again the fact that he feels the way he does and by negating again and again the conclusions to which his feeling state has led him — that his situation is hopeless, irreparable, and irrevocable. By offering him this support we can perhaps induce him to stand still long enough to take stock of his prison, to realize the nature of the bars in front of him, and to discover the existence of the open door behind his back.

The same general rule for interaction applies when a nurse works with bereaved persons, in individual instances or during a disaster. She should give credence to the state in which they find themselves, whether it is one of shock or denial, an uncontrollable urge to cry, or anger at the loved one for having abandoned them and left them with an almost unmanageable burden of responsibilities.

For the danger of grief does not lie in what one feels, but rather in one's inability to tolerate one's experience, one's thinking one should feel differently, one's blocking or repressing one's feeling state, one's consciously forbidding oneself to feel the way one does because one thinks it is not befitting to oneself or to the lost one. For the feelings, whether accepted or not, continue to lead their own existence − if necessary, outside one's awareness. Keeping them underground takes up one's energies; also they may suddenly burst forth at a most inopportune time, asking that the grief-work with them be continued. Here, just as in depression, the nurse must not be misled by the person's standards of conduct, but instead, must sustain him in what he does experience regardless of whether it is appropriate and acceptable. He does not have to give in to his experience if this seems inappropriate − that is, if he feels like laughing or crying or raging he need not necessarily do so − but it is all right for him to *feel* like it.

TERTIARY PREVENTION

How can nurses lessen impairment in those who have been in a state of grief or depression for a long time? The problem here, as I see it, is that people in this category do not seem to be grieving or depressed. Therefore, the first question is: How can the nurse recognize that such a person is in need of tertiary prevention? The answer lies in acquiring and utilizing knowledge about the symptomatology of grief and of depression, so vividly put forth in Dr. Thaler's article, There is denial; there is a feeling of emptiness; there is anger toward others and the self; there is self-pity. In depression there are feelings of hopelessness, worthlessness, and helplessness; there may be many somatic complaints.

Yet how frequently we nurses ignore the meaning of these symptoms! The long-term patient who acts as if his disease does not exist is likely to be categorized not as one who is denying the fact of his illness, but as "uncooperative." Angry patients are identified as "demanding" or "complaining," patients who frequently cry as "dependent," patients who feel hopeless as "resigned." The type of illness varies, but usually it is a long-term condition that has made a decisive difference in the patient's way of life — for example, diabetes, a coronary occlusion, arthritis, paralysis of one sort or another, or cancer. What is characteristic of all of these patients is that they cling tenaciously to their mode of behavior and seem unwilling to avail themselves of the rehabilitative services offered to them. Another common characteristic is that they are disliked by the nursing staff, who are frustrated by their stubbornness and their defeatist attitude.

What would happen if we nurses were to look at these patients from the viewpoint of what we know about grief and depression, if we were to consider them to be mired in one of the phases of grief and, instead of trying to push them into accepting their condition, an approach which has not helped them or us so far, were to acknowledge the fact that they can move neither backward nor forward in their attitude concerning their condition? What would be the result if the nurse were to indicate this insight on her part by acknowledging to such a patient that his present condition must be quite a change from what he has been used to? Such an opening might well be followed by a flood of statements by the patient that are congruent with the stage of grief in which he finds himself. He may completely ignore his present state, but talk for hours and hours about his various prowesses before he was ill. Or he may let loose with a barrage against the doctor whose intervention has made him, as he sees it, the wreck he is now. Or he may wallow in self-pity and count up all his life's losses as if he were reciting something he has learned by heart. Or he may say that he has never been any good, that his present condition is what he always knew would happen.

Here again it is important that the nurse not act prematurely and tell the patient that he has much to live for or that it is not the physician's fault he finds himself in his present state. Instead, she should let him take all the time he needs to move from one stage of the grief process to the next. To hurry him is to no avail, for before he has reached the final stage he will not let himself be rehabilitated anyway. Moreover, who can gauge the time required for him to integrate an extremely threatening and painful experience?

I venture the opinion that the majority of the patients to whom we have given this or that label are arrested somewhere in their grief-work. I further believe that if we nurses give them the opportunity to express their grief, regardless of the stage in which they are, they will start moving from that stage to the next, and then to the next. And if they live long enough and we have the patience, they will eventually reach the final stage of restitution, where they are able to accept their condition and to live with it and make the best of it in light of the help available to them.

There may be exceptions to this optimistic prediction, particularly among patients suffering from cancer, since in all likelihood they have been in despair about themselves most of their lives. Their illness has probably not caused their despair, but it is possibly an outcome of it. Perhaps, to convey to them in many direct and indirect ways that we care, that we expect nothing of them which they cannot give, will bring them some relief, some respite in their eternal self-condemnation. Perhaps it won't.

Here again, we can only offer our support and our "thereness." Some patients will be able to make use of it, others may not be willing or able to do so. But, at least, by accepting their subjective experience, we will not put them in the position of having to defend themselves against demands we made on them by virtue of our good intentions.

An office nurse might well find opportunities to help families with grief avoid depression. List the actions an office nurse could take to find out a mother's feelings (Dr. Ujhely's first example), and how she is coping during the critical period of her loss.

What is the meaning of "abreact"? How does it relate to unfinished grief-work?

Where does the *danger of grief* lie, according to Ujhely? How can a nurse help?

What comment was made about how earlier losses in a person's life affect his reaction to a present loss?

List some opening statements you might make to help a patient with symptoms of depression move forward or backward instead of being locked in to his depressed state—to help him with his grief work?

Open-ended conversation and listening are still major components of the nursing process. You may wish to review articles 6 and 13.

24.

The Coping Behaviors of Fatally Ill Adolescents and their Parents

June S. Lowenberg

In the previous articles, you have learned about the behavior of dying people and behaviors of those close to the person dying or suffering some loss. This article will help you organize your observations so that you will learn to recognize combinations of behaviors instead of being satisfied with isolated glimpses that could lead to inaccurate conclusions.

To establish a framework for understanding coping behavior, the definition used by Friedman et al. is useful: "Coping behavior is a term that has been used to denote all of the mechanisms utilized by an individual to meet a significant threat to his psychological stability and to enable him to function effectively." The behavior observed in response to threat is viewed as representing physical and psychological activity aroused to ward off anticipated danger.

When the fatally ill patient is a child or an adolescent the anticipation of death has a traumatic impact upon the parents as well, with consequent disruptive effects on family functioning. Because of the maximal intensity of the mother-child relationship, the fatally ill child poses a symbolic threat of death to the mother. A fatal disease that entails a number of remissions and relapses, such as leukemia or Hodgkin's disease, has an especially strong emotional impact on the stricken child and his parents.

In this discussion coping behaviors will be separated into two categories: (1) approach behaviors, which are aimed at coping with the realities at hand, and (2) avoidance (denial) behaviors which are directed toward the existence of these realities.

Avoidance mechanisms and their resultant patterns of behavior can be viewed as having either a positive or negative effect on the individual's adaptation. From the positive point of view, they are seen as protective measures that allow the individual to continue to function while faced with a major threat. In this sense, the mechanism is adaptive in that it enables the individual to remain fairly comfortable and to continue daily activities without serious disruption. In a situation where the threat cannot be realistically alleviated, the denial may be an appropriate way of coping with the threat.

On the other hand, to work through their relief , the patient and his family must abandon denial and avoidance mechanisms at least partially. In long-term fatal illness, the patient and his family may do a great deal of the grief work in advance of the actual death. This anticipatory work allows the patient to accept the inevitability of his own death and enables the family to go through the mourning process more rapidly than is possible when death is sudden and unexpected.

To provide appropriate emotional support to fatally ill patients and their families, nurses need more explicit tools for assessing where the patient and family are in the grief process. From observations of fatally ill adolescents and their families with whom I have worked, augmented by data recurring in the literature, I have compiled two lists of behavior indices, one of which includes manifestations of avoidance coping and the other manifestations of approach coping. The behaviors listed under this latter category are most often utilized by individuals who have at least partially abandoned avoidance and denial mechanisms and are moving through the process of grieving.

BEHAVIORAL INDICES OF COPING PATTERNS

AVOIDANCE BEHAVIOR

(Denying or Avoiding the Reality Situation)

Hostility toward physicians, nurses, other staff members

Intellectualizing and questioning about details of disease unrelated to the present condition (generalized information)

Avoiding discussion of death and related subject even out of context of the specific situation

Avoidance of staff; missed appointments

Parents' avoidance of patient

Overactivity without sense of loss (feelings of well-being)

Exhibiting no affect or expression of feeling while discussing diagnosis, prognosis

Psychosomatic symptoms

Progressive social isolation

Self-punitive behavior, such as expression of feelings of worthlessness

Behavior indicating magical thinking or excessive fantasy

Talk of unrealistic plans for the distant future

Behavior indicating that religion is being turned to increasingly

Focusing on minor complaints

APPROACH BEHAVIOR
(Working toward Acceptance, Restitution)

Focusing on the present condition of patient

Planning for the time of death and afterward

Asking questions about or discussing death and anticipated problems

Crying; expressing feelings of sorrow

Acknowledgement by parents that the child is aware of the situation

Somatic distress; restlessness

Withdrawal from social contacts; depression

Reviewing past and family relationships and experiences

Behavior indicating correct cognitive perception of the situation and search for new, appropriate knowledge

Seeking and utilizing help from both personal and institutional resources, including family gathering

Behavior indicating that religion is being turned to increasingly

Verbalizing one's nonacceptance earlier in the disease progression

In presenting these lists I wish to emphasize several points. First, they represent a beginning assessment tool only; as more data in this area are collected, the items in the list should be refined. Secondly, none of the indices can be used alone to indicate the type of coping patterns used by the individual. However, a combination of behaviors in one of the categories considered in the context of the entire assessment of the patient and his family should enable the nurse to judge fairly accurately the type of coping pattern involved. Assessment of this kind must be continually re-examined so that the movement of the patient and the members of his family can be noted and the nursing approach adjusted to their current situation.

Then, because of the complexity of human motivation and behavior, any of these behaviors can have differing implications depending on their context and the particular meanings ascribed to them by the individual. Among these ambiguous items are somatic distress, increasing dependence on religion, and hostility toward the medical and nursing staff.

Somatic distress may be an indication that the patient or the family member is involved in the work of mourning and therefore is beginning to work toward acceptance. On the other hand, strong denial over a period of time with failure to go through the grief process has sometimes been found to result in psychosomatic symptoms. The length of time since the diagnosis might give the nurse an indication of the coping pattern being utilized. It is obvious, also, that the patient's somatic distress could be a physiological result of the disease process or be related to other variables in the environment such as early viral infection. To use this index of behavior effectively, the nurse needs more than one observation, further knowledge about the patient and the length of his illness, and other behavioral signs.

The implications of increasing dependence on religion must be determined in the light of its meaning to the individual. Is prayer resorted to as a means of bringing about improvement and recovery (magical thinking) or is it a source of strength to the individual in facing the reality situation?

Hostility directed against staff can also be a manifestation of either avoidance or approach coping. Hostility of this type is commonly described in the literature discussing the early stages of grief during which the loss or anticipated loss is denied. On the other hand, hostility against physicians and nurses may be expressed during the terminal phases of illness when the patient or family has avoided facing the idea of death throughout the illness and suddenly realizes that death is approaching; in this instance, movement from nonhostile to projected hostile behavior would indicate a decrease in denial. Again, other variables must be considered in validating the supposed meaning of the manifestations. The family might have a reality-based complaint relating to neglectful care, and this perception could evoke the hostility.

The way in which the indices of approach-avoidance coping can be used to identify where a family is in relation to the grief process is illustrated by the following:

During the period immediately after Mr. and Mrs. F. had been told that their 13-year-old son, Douglas, had acute lymphocytic leukemia, they appeared to accept the diagnosis and prognosis. They spoke very matter-of-factly about the diagnosis with minimal or no affect and continually asked questions related to technical aspects of the disease while re-fraining from questions related directly to their son. Following the first lapse, the father asked the same questions repeatedly in what the physicians interpreted as a demanding manner; he also called the physician in charge of care repeatedly within a two-week period and went to another physician, who also requested validation from the first physician. The medical staff expressed surprise at the behavior because they viewed these parents as having completely accepted the diagnosis earlier. The medical staff withdrew from the parents and expressed feelings that Mr. and Mrs. F. did not realize how much they were trying to do for their son.

At the time of the first relapse the parents also insisted that Doug was unaware of the severity of the situation, despite his remarks to them that indicated he realized what was in store for him — for example, "You mean *if* I go home."

During the next remission both parents were friendly during clinic appointments. However, when I spoke to them alone one month into remission, they expressed disappointment that the first remission had been shorter than they had anticipated. They asked fewer questions, and those they asked were directly related to Doug's present condition and treatment. While Mrs. F. cried softly, Mr. F., almost in tears himself, stated that they were sure Douglas was aware of the severity of his illness.

Although the behaviors exhibited by Mr. and Mrs. F. prior to the first relapse might at first glance appear to indicate their acceptance of the reality situation of their son's illness and its outcome, their behavior was initially an attempt to deny and reverse the diagnosis while displaying intellectual acceptance. The two most important clues to their use of emotional denial were, first, the minimal stress or affect apparent while they were discussing the disease, and second, the numerous questions about aspects of the disease that were unrelated to their son's condition. From this information it could have been predicted that when their son relapsed they would probably react strongly. By the next remission their behavior showed more indication of approach patterns of coping and the beginning of anticipatory grief work: they displayed emotion appropriate to anticipatory grief work, asked questions more related to Doug's condition, and were able to see that Doug was aware of the severity of the situation.

Once the nurse understands how the fatally ill adolescent and his family are attempting to cope with the threat of death, she is faced with the problem of determining the goal of her interventions in relation to their coping patterns. Should she support avoidance tendencies, or should she endeavor to help the individual to initiate or move more rapidly toward approach behavior?

The main rationale for support of avoidance tendencies is based on their protective function. Because impending death is such a major threat, facing it may lead to intolerable and overwhelming anxiety. The individual and his family may be unable to function for an extensive period of time if avoidance mechanisms are taken away early in the course of disease.

On the basis of my studies, I believe that intervention aimed at altering denial is desirable only in carefully evaluated circumstances. If the nurse finds that a denial approach is being used, I believe she should attempt to alter this pattern of coping only if it severely impairs necessary functioning. For example, if parental denial results in their completely withdrawing a child from medical help, I would attempt to alter their cognitive perception of the reality situation. Or if the child or adolescent was in the process of dying and the parents maintained almost complete denial, I would attempt to alter their denial so that they could begin anticipatory grieving before their child's death.

Sixteen-year-old Steven C, the oldest of six children, died of Hodgkin's disease nineteen months after the disease had been diagnosed. His behavior during various points in his illness illustrates the progression of an adolescent from the avoidance-denial pattern to the approach pattern of coping.

During the period between April and June of 1968, approximately a year after diagnosis, Steven consistently exhibited the following behavior. He spoke at length about his illness, but without affect. He frequently verbalized feelings of worthlessness, speaking of himself as "not a whole man" and a "freak." Throughout this period of time, he showed minimal expression of feelings or emotions.

In the first four weeks of his last hospitalization he continued to verbalize about himself as a "freak", but with increasing affect. He began to focus on the details of his present condition, asking many questions which were oriented to the reality situation. He mentioned a study he had read that reported a 70 percent "cure" for Hodgkin's disease. During the second week of the hospital experience, he asked an orderly, "Why do I have these?", pointing to erupted surface nodes. During this same period, several times he accused the physicians of "giving up." He was able to express his anger both verbally and nonverbally, but often apologized afterwards. He began speaking at length about his family and friends and how he missed the ocean. He expressed guilt and fear that his mother had deserted him because he was unworthy. At other times, he said she didn't visit him because it hurt her so much and that she did care. Magical thinking was expressed fairly frequently along with less frequent references toward the future. He was able to seek and use help from his parents and staff during this time and would have nurses call his family and friends when he wanted visitors. At one point he asked me to write a letter to his next oldest brother, who was about to return home from several months' stay at a juvenile hall, in which he passed on to him the responsibility for the other siblings. He told him that he had faith in the brother's ability to "make good." He also expressed, with feeling, his sense of missing him and the other children.

During the last week preceeding his death, Steven increasingly spoke of death and his wish to die. He told me and the other staff members that if we wouldn't let him die he would have to find a way himself. After this statement, he refused food, saying that it would only make things last longer. He cried frequently, verbalizing his inability to "take it" any more and hating to be so helpless. He asked me to help by getting him some poison so that he could end his life faster. No matter how much time I spent with him, he asked me to remain, begging me not to leave. For the first time in the nine months of our association, he expressed feelings to me of some personal meaning in the relationship, telling me to "take care" whenever I left.

Two days before he died (the last day he remained oriented and alert except for one brief period immediately before death), when I said goodbye and told him when I would see him the next morning, he replied that he might not see me (this was stated very calmly, looking directly at me). We talked about the possibility that this might be a goodbye although I felt I would see him again. Just before a peaceful death, he did say his goodbyes to his family, to two other staff members, and to me.

Mrs. C, Steven's mother, used avoidance coping patterns during almost the entire period of her son's illness. She did not accompany Steven to the clinic. When I called to ask her to come in to see how Steve was doing, she came but stayed in the waiting room. When I approached her, she talked freely but without affect about its being "all Steve's problem," stating that he had to work it out for himself. She asked no questions directly concerned with her son's condition but expressed anger at the physicians, saying, "Some of them shouldn't be allowed to practice." When I asked if she had spoken to the social worker, she replied that the social worker "wasn't any help" and "couldn't communicate anyway."

Although Mrs. C's avoidance coping behavior allowed her to function in other areas, it impeded her functioning in relation to Steven. Part of his sense of wothlessness stemmed from her withdrawal from him, and his feeling of isolation during his final hospitalization was based on her absence. The general attitude toward Mrs. C on the part of the medical and nursing staff was one of hostility. Her functioning in relation to Steven was seen as more important than her defense against anxiety. She was seen as a "bad mother."

Initially I, too, reacted with inward hostility toward Mrs. C, but I thought her behavior worth investigating. In discussing Mr. and Mrs. C's previous coping patterns with the social worker, I learned that they were now separated and that both of them were alcoholics. I realized then that they habitually employed avoidance behavior to deal with stressful situations. Although their behavior deviated greatly from the normal expectations of the staff members, Steven had lived with it all his life.

These parents resisted all attempts to alter their behavior and at this point appeared unable to tolerate the stress that an approach coping pattern would activate. The hostility that Mrs. C expressed toward the social worker and the physicians and the fact that she avoided them also indicated that she would resist attempts to change her denial. I therefore focused my efforts on Steven and did not attempt to move Mrs. C away from avoidance coping. However, I watched closely for any change in her behavior that would indicate her readiness to move toward acceptance of the real situation.

Such an indication came when Mrs. C visited Steven one night ten days before he died. Steven was extremely depressed and had deteriorated physically since her last visit. I observed Mrs. C sobbing with her face turned away from Steven and holding onto his arm. I supported this early indication of grief work, attempting to show my availability for support without making demands. Since hitherto I had engaged in only superficial communication with Mrs. C, I did not talk to her but attempted to show my concern by silently offering her tissues.

When, two evenings later, Mr. and Mrs. C came while I was assisting Steven with his menu, I expressed my genuine pleasure at seeing them, again without making demands or inducing guilt over their past behavior. Then I asked Mrs. C if she wanted to help Steven to decide on the menu since she knew so much more about his food likes and dislikes than I did. The purpose of this intervention was to involve Mrs. C in Steven's care and to show her the alternate responses open to her which might provide satisfaction. It was also intended to show recognition of her unique value to Steven. This was an attempt at reinforcing her approach behavior.

Later interventions aimed at supporting Mrs. C's approach pattern included:

1. Interventions aimed at giving her some slight satisfaction to counterbalance all the stresses she was exposing herself to by being there. When she remained with Steven for long periods of time and appeared to become agitated, I would suggest that she needed a break. During breaks I spoke to her about how hard this must be on her and commented on the strength she was showing. These interventions were also aimed at relieving the guilt she expressed about not visiting Steven earlier in the course of the disease.

2. Interventions aimed at aiding her to go through the process of anticipatory mourning so that she would be prepared for the actual death insofar as was possible in the short time available. I allowed her to talk about the impending loss and its meaning to her. When I commented on how hard this must be for her, she began talking about how handsome and active Steven had been, and I encouraged her to talk about the way she remembered him and the differences now.

3. Interventions aimed primarily at reducing her guilt, since too large a burden of guilt would hinder the successful resolution of the grief process, and any further guilt would probably result in less ability to function effectively in caring for Steven's siblings in the future. When she spoke about how people thought she was horrible for not visiting Steven earlier and said that she could not take it before she realized he really was dying, I told her that I thought I could understand her reaction and the pain. I reassured her that Steven knew she cared

about him, repeating his comment that he knew she could not come because she cared too much.

4. Interventions aimed at letting her know she was not completely isolated in facing the situation. In these efforts I made use of nonverbal gestures and touch. When, during the two nights before Steven's death she cried and Mr. C did not offer support, I put my arm around her and stood by her and offered her tissues.

When I evaluated these interventions, using the behavioral indices for coping behaviors, the effects appeared to be positive. From the onset of my interventions Mrs. C exhibited increased approach behavior. She began visiting daily and remained with Steven almost constantly the last two nights before his death. She began to go through anticipatory grieving and, after his death, she was able to continue with the grief work. She wrote me two letters in the year following Steven's death, expressing the grief and pain she was experiencing. She was also able to call upon both the social worker from UCLA and the protective case worker* after her son's death. It must be remembered, however, that other variables influenced this change: Steven's increasing physical deterioration made denial more difficult; the social worker was working more closely with the family during this period and a protective case worker was seeing Mrs. C in the home; and as Steven's death approached Mr. C applied more pressure on Mrs. C to mobilize her resources. Because of these variables, it is extremely difficult to determine the extent of the benefit from my interventions. However, it is doubtful that Mrs. C would have moved as rapidly toward approach patterns of coping had the nursing staff continued to reject her.

This example, it is hoped, will illustrate how the theory pertaining to coping mechanisms can be applied in work with fatally ill children and their parents and how the behavioral indices can be used to guide intervention and to identify change due to the intervention. However, it should be emphasized that the indices should be viewed as guidelines rather than directives.

---

*A social worker who follows a family by court order when there has been evidence of child neglect.

If you have a situation available now, try to use the lists of behaviors. It is a resource that you will need to refer to when such patients are in your care. It is unrealistic to expect to remember all the behaviors unless you are working with such patients regularly. Remember where this list is and refer to it when needed. Also, think about sharing it with hospital personnel.

How did the nurse assist Mrs. C to face her crisis event and work through her feelings? Will Mrs. C be more or less prepared to face future crisis events and react in a healthy manner? Why?

WORKING
IT THROUGH

25.

Elderly Diabetic Amputees

Helen M. Arnold

The previous three articles have discussed the grief process and why it is important to recognize that a crisis even has occurred, and how people can be helped to grieve in a healthy manner. The next seven articles will give you more explicit patient situations in which to apply this knowledge.

Look for attitudes of diabetic patients who have faced amputation.

I interviewed 20 elderly patients who had lost a limb from diabetic gangrene and also talked with the nurses in charge of these patients' wards in a large chronic disease and convalescent home in order to get some background about them. The following are the themes that I saw emerge; they seem congruent with the findings of other, related studies.

GRIEF

After amputation is an established fact, one of the first tasks that the patient will have to face is the resolution of the grief he feels for his lost body part and function.

At this stage in the patient's recovery and rehabilitation, the nurse is of the most help to him if she is available to listen to him, to encourage the expression of his feelings about his loss, and to support him in his grieving process. The patient needs to realize that he has a right to feel sorrow and anger about his loss.

Closely related to how the patient views himself is the way he interprets others' view of him, particularly his close friends and immediate family. If he has been someone on whom others have depended, it will probably be a bitter and hard adjustment for him to accept not only his changed role, but also the attitudes toward it that the important others in his life will have.

HELPLESSNESS

The diabetic amputee has many fears. These include a fear of death, a fear of pain and incapacitation, and a fear that his disease will progress. The fear was demonstrated in more than a few patients by an "acceptance" of their misfortunes that did not seem to ring true. Instead, they gave the impression of being afraid to voice complaints about their fate. There were many statements like, "Some people are worse off. I can't complain," "If I can just sit here and crochet, I won't complain," and, "I don't worry about it—it was God's will." It seemed as though they were afraid to complain lest they suffer even more as punishment for their complaints.

Realistically, he *is* much less able or competent than he was when he had his legs, but the fear that he may be abandoned may cause him to appeal to others' sympathies by demonstrating that he is completely helpless.

The patient who feels overwhelmed by helplessness needs assistance in accepting the real limitations of his abilities and help in gaining some feeling of competence in using his remaining abilities to their utmost. This will be difficult at times because it is often easier, quicker, and more economical to do things *for* the patient than to wait the amount of time he requires to do the task himself.

The patient who remains in a state of feeling helpless in coping with his own life may come to view dependence as his only possible life style. The lives of many diabetic amputees seem to revolve around a dependence-independence conflict. For example, when interviewing patients that I would place in this particular category, I noticed that they talked with pride of their various independent accomplishments—such as being the president of the patients' fishing club, crocheting and designing baby clothes, going to grandchildren's homes—and yet in the next sentence they would emphasize their necessary and complete dependence on others.

Helpful nursing care and support in this conflict of the diabetic amputee would concentrate on the patient's positive accomplishments and treat the necessary dependence in a matter-of-fact way that would deemphasize it.

In addition to the way the individual patient adapts to stressful situations, there is another important factor that will determine the diabetic amputee's recovery and rehabilitation. One study of elderly patients who have had a lower leg amputation showed that depression was more pronounced in those who, preoperatively, had viewed the surgery as a cure-all for their physical complaints.

They had also tended to deny, preoperatively, the realistic limitations that amputation would impose upon their activities. In this same study it was also found that the loss or "death" of a body part seemed to symbolize to the older patient the imminent approach of his total death.

HOPELESSNESS

The prolonged depression that has become ingrained and that has settled into hopelessness and apathy presents a most difficult problem to both the patient and the nurse. When the patient has reached this state he will have little or no motivation to become rehabilitated. He has learned to use apathy or a lack of feeling as a defense against the feeling of pain, and he is not eager to give it up.

This is a frustrating problem for the nurse who attempts to help him reach a goal that he has convinced himself he does not want to reach. If the nurse does not accept the fact that her patient may be almost completely lacking in motivation, she may try to push the patient too much toward what is really her own goal. At this time, patience, waiting, and availability should be the main ingredients in the nursing care plan. If the nurse is able to be available at the right times, it is possible that the hopeless, apathetic patient might begin to take the first, tentative step out of his present deteriorated psychologic state.

However, it is also important that the nurse not assume that the hopeless patient has indeed given up for all time. This hopeless attitude on the part of the nurse will not help to keep her available to the patient who is far too dispirited to begin any change completely on his own. Instead, it will gradually lead to a situation where the nurse takes the patient's lack of motivation for granted and where she tends to give her limited time to other, more receptive patients. She eventually withdraws from the apathetic patient and then he is indeed in a hopeless state, with very little chance of receiving the help he needs to change. This point is particularly significant to nursing because it is the nurse who is frequently the last outpost of professional help that is available to him.

GUILT

The diabetic amputee is very often guilt-ridden, and this can greatly affect his rehabilitation. He may feel guilty because he thinks he might have taken better care of his feet and legs when he had them. Many of the diabetic amputees to whom I talked had an almost defensive attitude about the care they had taken of their feet and about their dietary regimens, past and present. Even if a diabetic were most conscientious in his dietary observances and in foot care, the fact that the regimen he followed obviously was not successful in preventing the loss of his limb is certain to make him doubt his own efforts and to feel somehow guilty.

An explanation of the inevitability of the arteriosclerotic process might help alleviate some of the guilt associated with past self-care, but it might also add to the patient's fears. Most of the patients appeared quite fearful, and it is possible that detailed explanations of a chronic, progressive disease would frighten many of them to an extent that would overbalance any relief from guilt that would be gained.

The diabetic amputee may also feel guilty because of his changed body image and self-image. I believe that these feelings of insecurity about their own self-images were what prompted many of the patients I interviewed to display their stumps to me. It was as though they were trying to gain reassurance and acceptance of themselves the way they *now* saw themselves to be.

In my interviews with diabetic amputees, I did discover something surprising. Only one patient—one whom I cared for myself over a span of several weeks—expressed any feelings of anger toward his surgeon, the physician who treated him before he developed gangrene, the staff in his present environment, or toward society or even fate in general. The reason these patients did not complain or express resentment was that they had given up hope: they considered that they already "had one foot in the grave"—for them, the cliche had become reality—and they had resigned themselves to death.

SENSORY RESTRICTION

And finally, the effect of extreme modification in the individual's mobility imposes a great deal of sensory deprivation on these people, which results in diminished drives and expectancies. The great reduction in mobility that follows amputation can also greatly diminish one's ability to interact. I feel that this last point contains one of the most important implications for the nursing care of the diabetic amputee. This particular patient needs desperately to experience an environment beyond his bed, his wheelchair, his room and, if possible, beyond his home. His verbalization of this need for increased mobility and sensory variation may take a very direct form. Among the comments made by patients I talked to: "I have nothing to do here but wheel my chair in the hall, I'm stuck here!" and, "I only wish I could see New York City again—but I can't travel, so I never will."

The plea for help may be voiced in a much more subtle manner, such as, "Every day is the same as the last around here," or, as one patient said, "You can hear screaming and talking—people with their minds almost gone—they should put these people someplace else: it's not good to listen to, and I *have* to be here whether I like it or not!"

When it is not possible for the patient to be physically mobile beyond his present environment, he should be encouraged to be psychologically mobile—through interests, hobbies, current events, interpersonal relations—beyond his present environment. Sensory variation could also be obtained by enriching the scope of his interpersonal contacts through encouraging staff members to spend even brief periods talking with the patient about events outside of the hospital.

The ways and means of helping to vary the sensory environment of the severely restricted individual are limited only by one's creativity and imagination, and it is in areas such as this that the practice of nursing can be experienced as an art.

Compare the suggested nursing actions for the problem of hopelessness and apathy of the diabetic amputees in this article with the nursing actions for depressed patients in the next article "Cues to Interpersonal Distress Due to Pregnancy."

26.
Cues to Interpersonal Distress
Due to Pregnancy

Anthony R. Stone

*What does ambivalence mean to you? What are some signs of
ambivalence, rejection, or acceptance that you recognize in
everyday conversation? What recent occurrence has caused you
to have mixed feelings? Read the following article with the idea
of finding signs of ambivalence.*

The moment of confirmation of pregnancy can be considered dramatic for all
women, whether they are married in the formal sense or not; whether it is the
first, third, sixth, or nth; whether it was part of the family plan or not.

Intermeshed with every woman's own personal drama is another which is
found in the reactions she creates within her tiny segment of society, her family.
Her open and subtle indications of acceptance, ambivalence, or rejection of her
condition inevitably stir up responses and repercussions among her family
members, relatives, and friends.

In pregnancy, as with any major physiologic change such as adolescence,
there are certain built-in disruptive factors which may be defined as "temporary
impairment of an individual's usual capacity to cope with changing environmental stresses. . .often accompanied by heightened states of physical tension
and unpleasant affective reactions. These reactions include depression, grief,
resentment, worry, anxiety. . . .

Amid caring for the "normal" stresses indigenous to pregnancy, which must
be handled, one may often lose sight of the expectant mother's subtle or even

open indications of ambivalence or rejection of the reality of her condition. To the keenly sensitive care-giver, however, such perceived indications may provide important cues revealing need for more than routine attention by outside experts, if family equilibrium is to be maintained.

FAMILY AS A SOCIAL SYSTEM

While all members are important, it can be assumed that the father of the child-to-be retains the highest level of importance for the pregnant woman. Thus, the nurse may open pathways for the patient to comment about how the father-to-be and the children are reacting to the pregnancy.

Actually, even in the best of circumstances, where the mother and father claim to have planned for the pregnancy and appear eagerly to anticipate the new arrival, there are certain changes in family structure which have to be accepted and accomplished before effective interdependent familial patterns can be re-established and maintained.

Acceptance of the pregnancy, even if fatalistic in tone, is the prescribed cultural norm.

Ambivalence can almost always be counted as present. These mixed feelings are not often communicated spontaneously to other family members, including the husband. But, on probing by the recognized care-giver, these feelings may be laid on the table. In that process of opening up, they become that much less devastating.

The pregnant woman's world may be one of clashing values which storm beneath her mask of outward calm. She may be deeply concerned about the apartment regulations which "allow" only two children, while this pregnancy is her third. The vacation that had to be postponed may be her burden of guilty resentment. The family car that has to be kept for an indefinite time with all its needed repairs and general upkeep may be the concern through which her husband indirectly expresses his harassment. Her club and voluntary association activities which provide some status and fulfillment may have to be curtailed. The family budget may have to be stretched. Her own occupational success and its financial and status and other rewards may have to be put aside. All these things are important sources of stress deep in her secret heart as she and her family plod through the steps that lead to delivery. It is rare that a woman is immune from them. It is equally rare that she has a routine opportunity to discuss them with someone who understands.

NURSE AND THE PATIENT

In the patient's opinion, the nurse may be the key care-giving figure. The patient may pray for the opportunity to discuss personal matters with her. She may be the one person in whom the patient feels she can confide with immunity and with womanly empathy. Also, the nurse may be the key person on whom others in the constellation of experts available to the becoming mother may depend for basic information concerning the progress of the expectant mother. Unfortunately, it is often the clearly physiologic progress that preoccupies those caring for the pregnant woman. . .

Neither the nurse nor the obstetrician, for that matter, is expected to be a psychotherapist in the strict sense. But, together, they may provide a unique source of human warmth and understanding based on unique opportunities for observation based on physical care. Let us consider some of the sources of such cues which may be readily available to nurses.

The first obvious sign which may be picked up by the nurse may be excessive delay in the patient's making contact with appropriate prenatal, care-giving services. Did she attempt to keep her condition secret through use of constricting garments? Does she deny that the pregnancy was possible and hope for some other diagnosis, ominous as such alternative might be? The woman who waits until the fourth or fifth month is clearly in some sort of conflict about her role in pregnancy.

Then, there is the case of the woman who runs to her obstetrician a day after a delayed menstrual period. Or the one who is so sure she is pregnant that she seeks out nursing counsel long before there is sufficent evidence. In general, excesses in feelings are danger signs. Excessive joy, excessive fear, excessive secrecy, nausea, pain, bleeding, demands for sick role status, excessive casualness about returning to work in a week or so after delivery, and all the rest cannot, or should not be, ignored by the nurse in charge. Also, blame of husband or self must be noted and discussed, as with excessive rumination about the probabilities of delivering an abnormal child. Excessive discussion and even reported arguments about the expected sex of the coming infant or even the name to be chosen should be noted.

SOME INDICATORS OF CONFLICT

The basic history contains many cues for the nurse with whom the newly pregnant woman has made contact. First of all, is there evidence that the patient has experienced emotional problems during her lifetime? That is, has it been necessary for her to seek psychiatric or psychologically oriented counseling help before? More important, if formerly pregnant, has she a history of attempted induced abortion? Has it been years since her last pregnancy? Just a few months? These are sensitive subjects and require some intensive listening. Fifteen or 20 minutes on the nurse's part may pay off considerably in the treatment program for the woman. Discussion can be part of the routine antepartal care, even during such procedures as taking blood pressure or obtaining a urinalysis.

Listen for what the newly pregnant woman asks. Who is the person most referred to in conversation? The husband? Herself? The baby in her womb? The other children? Her mother? Whoever that person is, he is important. The nurse may find it most informative to ask about the patient's interactions with that person. This opportunity to pick up cues should not be missed.

A most important cue is generally conceptualized in terms of the pregnant woman's appraisal of the value of the pregnancy itself. She may think and talk of how useful the new baby will be to herself, the marriage, or to the siblings. The theme of, "having someone to love me," may be a danger sign. The theme of, "what this baby can do for us," is worth serious consideration. The moment the value of the expected infant is placed outside himself, the nurse must begin listening to the patient with her "third ear."

OTHER CUES TO CONFLICT

The "simple" fact of excessive nausea and pleading for invalid status with a tendency to make pregnancy into an illness beyond practical limits calls for special attention. Similarly, bragging about her own individual skill in becoming pregnant may be a danger sign. With these may go the minimizing of the husband-wife interactional roles.

Finally, in this country, the term, "just a housewife," has become common. The expecting woman who looks with derogatory feelings on what is "left" for her, once the baby arrives, is as vulnerable as any of those mentioned earlier. Sometimes, her comments about the nurse's professional status and role may provide cues to how she feels about what is ahead for her. If these things happen, what can the nurse do about it?

COUNSELING-REFERRING ROLE

As with the other cues, next to listening sympathetically, she can discuss some of the factual details with the patient, which may reveal leads about deeper conflict. Certainly, it takes some time. But who besides the nurse may be available for such counseling? Straightforward answers, plus reflecting techniques to help the patient find her own way out of her dilemmas, take some extra time. But the same amount of time could have been spent in discussing diets and taking blood pressure ad nauseam, because these were the easiest things to do and may have been what the patient seemed to want most.

But, with all this grist for her mill, what does the nurse who senses deep conflicts within the heart of her antepartal patient do to help beyond what she herself can offer in routine listening, reassurances, and physical ministrations? In the first place, she ought to discuss her evidence with the obstetrician in charge. Secondly, she ought to return to the patient with some orientation concerning specific problems which need to be handled. Thirdly, she should use her influence as a referring person. She might first contact the council of social agencies in her particular locality and discuss the needs of the case. As community resources and their specific functions are defined, the nurse should prepare herself for the task of helping the patient get to the appropriate agency or therapist for assistance with whatever problems seem to be concerning her. This could be an agency for families and children, a department of public welfare, a private-practicing marriage and family counselor, a private-practicing psychotherapist and, in some cases, a psychoanalyst.

In any case, the reasons for the referral and a discussion of the possible alternatives ought to be shared fully with the patient. As the decision is approached, it should be the patient who makes the final choice. Chances are that after the rather extensive and intensive contact with the antepartal nurse, a discussion about such matters will come easily.

What signs did you read about that could indicate rejection? Acceptance? Pride? Blame? Guilt? Talk with your mother, sister, aunt, or friend about her feelings about each pregnancy. Be ready to listen and look for cues.

What other ages have problems of ambivalence or conflict? Teenager? Toddler? Working mother? Parents with newly grown children? Retired persons? List at least two examples of situations that are likely to cause ambivalent feelings in the age groups listed above.

What guidelines did this article give the nurse that would also guide her actions in helping any of the above people with conflict?

27.
Milieu Design for Adolescents with Leukemia

Joel Vernick
Janet L. Lunceford

How would you feel if you were told that you would be caring for a youngster with a fatal illness? Could you handle the concerns of a seriously ill adolescent?

Since this article was written, progress has been made in the treatment of leukemia and some young patients with leukemia have gone into remissions that may be permanent. But until the treatment has been perfected to reach all patients, this article remains relevant.

Some persons might view a cancer nursing unit as one in which an atmosphere of dread and fear prevail. This atmosphere does not surround our twenty or more adolescent patients over a period of a year with leukemia on the Chemotherapy Service of the National Cancer Institute. Our program, milieu management, is similar to those developed in residential treatment of emotionally disturbed children.

Our program is based on the philosophy that the patient is helped more by being able to talk about his fears and anxieties and problems—including the possibility of death—than by dealing with these problems alone.

Anyone has difficulty responding to many questions that adolescents ask about their progress and their conditions, especially the question, "Am I going to die?" Our emphasis on frank discussion does not mean that we would give an affirmative answer to such a question. Rather, all professional workers in the unit are encouraged to offer children an opportunity to talk about the matters that worry them, and this includes death. At the same time, we stress that children should be told there is always hope and that the medical team is doing everything possible to get them well enough to return home.

The more a patient knows about his own condition and progress and those of his friends and other patients on the floor, the less anxious he becomes. Of course, all anxiety is not dissipated. But, our goal is the freeing of anxiety in as many areas as possible to enable the patients to function more productively.

FUN AND RESPONSIBILITIES

We are concerned with creating an atmosphere to meet, to the highest degree possible, the physical, emotional, and social needs of the patients. They themselves prefer to be treated as they were before they became sick.

The patient activities program provides weekly movies, Friday night bingo, traveling stage shows, gym activities, arts and crafts, band concerts, and the like. Occupational therapy is another program that provides varied activities to maintain maximum functioning of patients. Bedside programs are offered by occupational therapy where necessary. Children have many picnics and cookouts, go swimming at the local pools in the summertime, visit local points of interest, and make trips to the drug store.

INTERVIEWS WITH CHILDREN

The social worker holds individual and group interviews with the children. They discuss their feelings about their illness and decide how to discuss leukemia with their friends, relatives, and teachers. On rare occasions these group interviews are formally scheduled. The social worker is on the nursing unit for the entire working day and the nursing staff are also always available, giving children many opportunities for discussions with them. In addition, trips, while providing enjoyment for the children, also serve as occasions when all subjects are open for discussion.

When youngsters' questions about leukemia require the answers of a physician, we arrange for the chief pediatrician to meet with the patients.

When the social worker interviews a child or a group in a patient's room, it is understood (as discussed at weekly team meetings) that any nursing personnel who enter the room are welcome to become involved. The group might be discussing the death of a patient, and the social worker will say to the nurse, "We were just talking about Penny." This draws her into the discussion. The exchange during such interviews is therapeutic for all—staff and patients.

HELPING PATIENTS TALK

To free a patient to talk about himself, his friends, and death, staff members must understand the serious predicament of the patient. This is crucial. The best way to communicate this understanding is to answer questions truthfully. One can be friendly, cheerful, and cooperative, but this is not the same as helping the patient with the basic problems at hand—mainly, the fear of dying and death.

However, we recognize that all nurses cannot agree to or feel free to discuss such matters. Particularly at the outset of our program, there was much resistance. The general attitude expressed verbally and nonverbally was: The less these problems are discussed, the less upset the children will be. Also, some nurses thought milieu management would cost them time needed for physical care of patients.

We decided, therefore, that all nurses on the unit need not become involved. At one of the team meetings, the choice was put to the nursing staff as follows: Those who were willing to discuss such matters with the children could, and support would be provided for them. Those who wished to avoid such subjects were to inform a questioning child that someone else would talk with him, and then to tell the head nurse or the social worker the child had questions.

The more individual and group interviews the social worker held with the children, the more staff nurses could see that, contrary to their earlier belief, such action did not upset the patients. Rather, more healthful emotional functioning resulted. Gradually, some of the nursing staff adopted this approach. An important aspect of this process was the weekly team meetings and informal discussions, in which the social worker discussed interviews held with the children. Conferees focused their attention, not only on the problems of the children, but also on the difficulties of the staff in adapting to the problems.

Nurses also realized that the "extra" work was something that they could accomplish during such routine activities as giving medications and taking temperatures. As some staff members exhibited willingness to talk, patients were able to communicate more readily on a meaningful level.

It is interesting to note that the patients did not take our word about encouraging them to ask questions. They tested staff members. Rapidly, they determined which staff members would answer and which would be evasive or not tell the truth and they put all staff members in either of two categories. Thus, those on whom the patients knew they could rely for honest discussion were the ones with whom they established closer relationships.

DEATHS OF FRIENDS

Despite the diversions and activities that the hospital personnel provide, the adolescent never escapes from the omnipresent knowledge about leukemia and his impending death. He is with others who have the same disease from remission to the terminal state. He soon becomes sophisticated about the actions of the staff and the equipment associated with terminal care—the oxygen equipment, the hypothermia machine, and the electrocardiograph. He also knows that the patients nearest the nurses' station are usually the most seriously ill.

Nurse B. was in the nurses' station with the head nurse when C., aged 13, approached and asked if a certain patient had died. Miss B. became momentarily flustered. Afterward, she said, "It was very hard for me to answer the question. However, I was almost at once convinced that I should tell her the truth, and so I did."

Another patient, T., age 13, approached Miss V. and asked, "Did something happen last night?" Something had happened. T's friend had died.

One way to deal with such a round-about question is to feign a misunderstanding of the true question that is being asked. Miss V., however, revealed insight and sensitivity. She said, "Do you mean, did somebody die last night?" Then they discussed the impact of it on T.

While these are only two examples which indicate several stages of intellectual and emotional development when the stimulus for learning is present, many more could be cited. However, it also needs to be pointed out that there were those on the nursing staff who were unable to involve themselves in such an emotional area, and in the final analysis, each person has to resolve such problems in the manner best suited to his own intellectual and emotional adjustment.

Are you a staff member who would want to discuss these problems or avoid them? It is important to recognize your own position and to strengthen your skills in helping patients cope with impending death for their friends, family, and for themselves.

28.

The X Factor in Nursing

Norma J. Peters

*The x factor – you already know it by other names, and, hopefully,
you recognize it and cultivate it as you care for your patients.*

What is good nursing?

Everyone seems to be trying to define it in professional, philosophical,
psychological, educational, legal, or pragmatic terms, according to the viewpoint
of the definition writer. But can it be defined? Is there not an x factor present
that can only be shown by example in order to be meaningful?

I think there is. In nursing classes, I've found the four brief scenes described
here helpful in giving meaning to the x factor. Both student nurses in these
scenes are kind and skillful. They organize their work and try to help their
patients to the best of their ability. But only one of them makes use—
instinctively, perhaps—of the x factor. See if you can determine which nurse
does—Miss Smith, left column, or Miss Jones, right.

Here is the scene: The patient, Mr. Haddad, 49, has had a successful
commissurotomy for mitral stenosis. For several years his physical activity had
been greatly restricted because his heart couldn't supply the blood output
needed. Now all that lies behind him, though he doesn't realize this yet. He is
now in the final few days of hospitalization.

Nurse on morning visit

"Hi, Mr. Haddad, I'm Miss Smith. You
look good. Nice color—that's a good

Nurse on morning visit

"Hi, Mr. Haddad. I'm Miss Jones. How
are you?"

*From "The X Factor in Nursing" by Norma J. Peters, published in the July 1971
issue of* R.N. *Copyright © July 1971 by Litton Publications Inc. Reproduced,
with permission, from* R.N.

sign. I'll set up the water, and you wash your face and hands. O.K.?"

"All right, I guess."

"Good. You *look* good. You have nice color, and that means your circulation is good."

"The doctor says my heart's never been better."

"Wonderful! It must be a grand feeling. Listen, I'll put your water and mouthwash in front of you. Will you wash your face and hands?"

"Always do, and I'm glad to."

"Swell. I'll see you in a little while because I want to help my other patients."

Nurse returns

"All set? Let me change the water, and I'll wash you. So, what's new?"

"Not much. I'm not doing too much these days, you know."

"Uh-huh. But there's not too much to do around here anyway. Pretty soon you'll be running around and having a good time."

"Well, I get nervous about what I'll be able to do when I get home. You know what I mean?"

"Sure, but don't worry. The doctor will explain everything to you. He'll answer all your questions and you'll really be satisfied."

"I have so many questions—"

"Listen, don't worry. They'll all be taken care of. Just be patient."

"Yes, you're right, I guess."

"Sure I am. I'm your trusty nurse!"

Nurse returns

"All set now. I'll change the water and continue your bath. I bet you'll be glad when you can do the whole bath yourself. That'll be soon, too, because you're going home the end of the week. Isn't that good?"

"Yes, it is. I get nervous, though. I'm not sure what I'm going to do at home—how much I'll be able to do."

"Well, Mr. Haddad, Dr. Brown will never let you go home without a full explanation—written, too—of exactly what you'll be able to do. Really, he's very good about that. And one of us will be with him to explain further if you have any questions when he leaves. Let me put lotion on your feet. They're very dry. . . .You know, when you go home I think it'd be a good idea if a nurse came in once a week to see if everything is all right. The Visiting Nurse Association provides that service. A nurse could make things easier. You could sort of lean on her a little, you know. We could suggest it to Dr. Brown, and he would take care of it."

"That would be great! Just to have

her look in every so often would ease my mind. I know I'm all right and I'm really not afraid. It's just that home is different from here."

"Easily arranged. Fear not—we will manage all!"

Mrs. Haddad visits

"Hello, Mrs. Haddad. Well, he'll be going home soon. Bet you're happy."

"I certainly am. I'm trying to fix everything so it'll be easy for him. I wish I knew just what to do."

"Never mind. I know you must be doing a fine job. Keep it up. Good-bye now."

Mrs. Haddad visits

"Hello, Mrs. Haddad. Isn't it good your husband is going home?"

"It certainly is. I'm trying to fix everything in the house to make it easy. I wish I knew just what to do."

"You mean like where to sleep and eat to avoid a lot of unnecessary walking?"

"Yes, those things."

"Gee, Mrs. Haddad, wait a minute and I'll check on something that might help you." She leaves briefly, then returns. "Miss Considine, the head nurse, just spoke with Dr. Brown. He told her it would be all right to have a nurse from the Visiting Nurse Association come to your house before your husband comes home. She can help you with your planning. Would you like that?"

"Are you kidding? I'd love it! I'll pay her anything."

"I don't think they charge much, but I can check."

"No, no. It's all right. You've done more than enough, and I thank you very much."

"You're welcome. Have a good visit now."

Final dinner

"Hi again. Well, it's liver and onions so it must be Tuesday. Right?"

"Oh, God, I get sick on liver. I can't eat it, honest."

Final dinner

"Hi again. Well, pheasant under glass. In the form of liver and onions. O.K.?"

"Oh, God, I really can't eat liver."

"That's all right. I'll call and see if I

"Well, just eat the other stuff. This once will be O.K."

"Yes, but I'm really hungry."

"Oh, well, I guess I could call the kitchen. Boy, they'll yell; but don't you worry, I'll get you something else." Later: "Here's a steak—happy eating."

"Thank you."

can get you anything else. Would you like anything special?"

"I love steak."

"O.K." Later: "Here you are. Hope it's good."

"Thank you."

"We'll miss you, Mr. Haddad, but we're glad you feel so well. If I don't see you again, good luck."

"Thank you. You've been wonderful to me."

Do you have your answer ready? It's Miss Jones who demonstrates the x factor, isn't it? She knows more about her patient than Miss Smith and is more interested in him as an individual. She encourages him to express himself. She listens and hears and is *specifically* helpful.

The x factor is this: a warmth and a delight in life and all who are a part of life. Some call it *empathy*.

Write down your feelings and comments as you read each nurse's interactions. What do you think each is thinking or feeling? How do these compare with your own thoughts?

If you *really* want to be a nurse like Miss Jones, what specific steps can you take to proceed in that direction? List these steps.

What if, as a graduate, your hospital or unit is understaffed and you have little time and must delegate care to a nursing assistant? What happens to Miss Jones in that situation?

29.

Separation Anxiety

Jeanette Nehren
Naomi R. Gilliam

Think about the feelings you have when a special loved one is leaving from an airport or a railway station. Look around and you will see evidence of others with similar signs of separation anxiety. How do you cope? How can you help patients cope? This is what this section is all about. As you read, stop and relate comments in the article to your own feelings.

The termination of an interpersonal relationship can be a problem to any or all of us. The feelings we encounter when someone we treasure leaves us can cause a type of pain that cannot be relieved by a hypodermic injection, tranquilizer, or even a pleasant "good-bye."

We have noticed that if the nurse-patient relationship has been intensive or the patient's hospitalization has been extensive, both the nurse and the patient may experience feelings of loss when the patient is discharged or when the nurse leaves the nursing care unit. The feelings centering around this object loss may be expressed in many ways. Because of our cultural orientation, they are not likely to be verbalized and may not always be recognized.

Patient: Well, I'm all packed. I guess I'm ready to go now.

Nurse: Did you get your medicines from the pharmacy?

Patient: Yes.

Nurse: Check with the business office?

Patient: Yes.

Nurse: Yes, you are ready to go. I'll get an aide to help you with your luggage.

Patient: You have been very kind during my illness. I want to thank all of the nurses. I know I've been a difficult patient for you to handle.

Nurse: You've been here a long time. Let's see, it's been three months. Gee, I'll bet you will be glad to get home.

Patient: Yes. . .that's great I guess. (He smiles wanly and turns away. The nurse watches from the nursing station as he slowly walks down the hall.)

Every nursing practitioner has witnessed or participated in interactions similar to this one. How often do we stop to ask what is happening? Why is the patient so hesitant about leaving? Why does the nurse seem so interested in his medicines and business matters, but show so little interest in him? Why does she keep him from venting his feelings?

The phenomenon of separation anxiety was first identified by Freud in 1905. He related it to the reaction of the loss of a loved object and the pain of mourning. Otto Rank believed that separation anxiety first occurs at birth when an infant is separated from his mother but, according to Klein, a child first experiences separation anxiety at the time of weaning, thus creating in the child feelings of depression and persecution. . .

The degree of anxiety and depression created at early separation experiences will determine how the individual will manage future separations or termination of friendships during his entire lifetime. The love, security, and trust the mothering figure gives to the infant and young child at these crucial periods of emotional development help prevent feelings of rejection, depression, or guilt, and the need for punishment in future separations.

Probably another major separation experience by a child is separation from the family to the school and its significant people. Again in middle-class America the end of the teens usually is a time when separation from the family to college, a job, the military services, or to marriage occurs. In the healthy person, this is a time when dependency on parents ceases—a time when anxiety and depression may occur. An individual does not always move from one emotional developmental level to the next with adequate feelings of love, security, and trust from those persons who are significant to him at these particular times in his life. For instance, the loss, through death or divorce, of one or both parents during a crucial developmental stage of life may occur without love and support from another person. The loss of other significant persons in his life-teachers, classmates, and friends—may also affect a person's later capacity to manage separation anxiety. The sense of loss may be the same regardless of who does the leaving, and the loss may be perceived as a feeling of rejection, loss of a loved object, or the need for punishment.

The nurse seldom knows—nor is it important for her to know—all a patient's experiences of early separations from significant people. But, in order to understand a patient's feelings and behavior, she does need to know that his feelings are primarily a revival of feelings of earlier separations and terminations. These feelings transferred to her may be either conscious or unconscious. The nurse also needs to recognize her own feelings about a pending separation. Frequently, she may need help in identifying her own feelings and the manner in which she expresses them. A teacher, co-worker, doctor, or supervisor may help her do this. Such persons can provide an opportunity for her to express her feelings of anger or loss and help her relate her feelings to separation anxiety. Increased self-understanding may evolve which may help her to help the patient.

In order to cope with separation anxiety, both patient and nurse will utilize defense mechanisms which they have found useful in maintaining their self-esteem in past experiences. However, these unconscious responses to perceived or actual object loss may not always be effective under stress situations and the nurse can help the patient find other mechanisms for expressing his anxiety.

Theoretically, termination for the patient begins for him at the time of his first contact with the nurse, doctor, hospital, or community agency. At this time the staff should focus their health teaching upon the day when the patient no longer will be dependent upon them. For instance, when a nurse teaches a patient with diabetes to give himself injections, she is preparing him for the time when he must take care of himself.

Preparation for termination may not be the same for all patients. For example, a patient who has had an appendectomy and is hospitalized for five days will have different feelings about leaving the hospital than the patient with a chronic illness who has had a long hospitalization. As with other interpersonal relationships such specific variables as the physical or mental health of the patient, former separations, the person who is leaving, the intensity and length of the nurse-patient relationship, and the patient's current relationships in the family and the community determine the degree of anxiety present.

When a nurse structures a continuous relationship with a patient he is entitled to know what expectations the nurse has for him and what expectations he may hold for her. In the initial contact, she should tell him how often she will see him, the length of time she will stay with him, and how long she will be working with him. Many times the nurse does not know all these details in the beginning but she should keep the patient informed when she is able to do so.

A patient's initial response to being told that the nurse will be leaving him or that he is being discharged may be denial. This reaction may be a denial of the pending separation or a denial of any significance in the separation. It may be expressed in behavior or in words. If the patient can be helped to recognize the meaning of his behavior he may be able to manage a healthy resolution of the separation anxiety. The following example from a process recording shows a nurse confronting a patient who had denied that his nurse was leaving although he had been told several times that she would leave him.

Patient: I look at people as an accounting problem. Some of them are listed under credits or debits. If I like them and they seem to like me, they're an asset. If they don't like me, they're a liability. But the columns keep changing.

Nurse: If people you care for do something that you don't like, what happens then?

Patient: They go under the liability column.

Nurse: I will be leaving March 13. I wonder what kind of feelings you'll have about me.

Patient: Well, I won't commit suicide, if that's what you mean.

In the interaction the nurse again confronted the patient with the fact that she would be leaving. At this time, he could no longer deny the fact, but could deny its significance.

A nurse may also deny her feelings about the separation or deny her own importance to the patient. In doing so, she may prevent his expressing positive or negative feelings toward her. She may encourage him unconsciously to keep conversation on a superficial level. Failing to mention that she is leaving or failing to mention the patient's pending discharge exemplify her denial or repression.

A patient may be overwhelmed by a sense of hopelessness or helplessness when denial is no longer effective. Anger and hostility may be a means of coping with these feelings. The patient may be angry with the nurse for leaving him or may feel that she is making him leave. These feelings may be expressed in various ways. Anger may be directed toward the nurse but may be focused on some incident other than the termination. More often, the anger may be directed toward another member of the staff, his own family, or another patient. If an open display of anger is alien to the patient, he may resort to being late for appointments, attempting to terminate the nursing interview early, or telling the nurse how "good" other personnel treat him. Finally, the patient may make use of projection as a defense against his anger. He may perceive that the nurse or another person is angry with him.

The nurse who is aware of the dynamics underlying such anger will respond to the patient's feelings of hopelessness and helplessness by being supportive. Becoming angry with the patient only would reinforce his feelings of rejection. Accepting his behavior as something to be explored with him enables him to start resolving his anxiety. If the nurse is not able to cope with her own feelings related to the termination, she may respond with such forms of anger as forgetting promises to the patient, cutting down the amount of time she spends with him, or by including other patients in their conversation.

Withdrawal is another device which the patient may employ during the termination of a meaningful relationship. He may not keep appointments. He may not talk to the nurse or, if he does, he may keep the conversation on a very superficial level. Nurses also use this mechanism.

Frequently, the patient who is awaiting discharge has little contact with the nursing staff. Although the physical care needed at this time may be minimal, the patient's psychological discomforts may increase.

Separation anxiety may be so intense that regression occurs. The psychiatric patient may return to his delusional system. The surgical patient may experience pain and request his postoperative medication. The medical patient may have a recurrence of symptoms. The public health patient may telephone for another visit. The nurse may begin to feel guilty for leaving the patient or the doctor may reconsider the discharge order. Because of her guilt, the nurse may allow the patient to manipulate her. She may have set aside an hour to be with the patient, but may stay longer. She may ignore phases of the patient's behavior with which he would ordinarily be confronted; for example, breaking his diet. Failing to set limits may, as a matter of fact, increase the patient's anxiety and reinforce his dependency needs.

Recognizing that the resolution of separation anxiety is not a constant, ongoing process, the nurse should reinforce the healthy components of the patient's personality at this time. She should be consistent. She should continue to evoke the exploration of feelings, to point out the significance of relationships, and to teach mental health principles. She also should constantly remember that backsliding may occur in any termination process. The process which enables the patient to use the healthier features of his personality varies with each interpersonal relationship. It is dependent upon the treatment goals for the patient, his self-awareness, and his ego strength.

Although a patient may have shown infantile idiosyncrasies in the early stages of termination, often the healthier features of his personality are mobilized for the final leaving. The hospital environment does provide a measure of security and permits the expression of feelings on a regressed level. The outside world is less tolerant. Rationalization, a socially accepted defense mechanism, is an aid in preserving ego integration at this time. A surgical patient who had not been prepared for termination and had been informed of his pending discharge on the day prior to this interaction aptly demonstrated his ability to rationalize in the following:

Well, then it's O.K. So, today's the day, huh? I been thinking about it
and I figure I'll be better off at home, anyhow. Around my own things,
eat some good Italian food, and get my strength back. So, it's all for
the best. I'm ready to go at any time.

If she understands the psychodynamics of feelings in the termination of a meaningful relationship, the nurse, hopefully, can manage her own feelings, accept the patient, and guide him toward resolving some of his feelings during this critical time. The patient may feel rejected, hopeless, helpless, or worthless as he is faced with leaving or being left by someone who has listened, understood, accepted, and assisted him in solving his own problems in daily living conflicts. This separation, though, may well be a less painful experience than experiences he may have encountered earlier.

Listen to people who are taking their leave — note how superficial the conversations are. How do you think each one might react if a deeper level of conversation were started?

Role play assisting a person to relate to another person instead of to a nurse.

Have you known patients whose conditions became worse as discharge neared? A patient with a new colostomy develops diarrhea or has a skin problem that requires longer hospitalization. A patient with heart disease develops chest pain and insomnia before discharge. A new mother develops mastitis. List some specific ways you can help these patients prepare for their discharge and summon up their own inner strengths.

How is separation anxiety related to the grief reaction? When does preparation for terminating a relationship begin and how does a nurse manage it?

30.

The Case for Parent-Child Nursing

Constance Nissen

If your child had to be hospitalized before he reached the age of six, at which age would you most prefer it to occur and why? Would you wish to stay with him 24 hours a day? Why or why not?

How does a child's behavior change when he is separated from his home and family?

Since 1951, a number of studies have shown that separating the young child from his parents during hospitalization may cause extreme anxiety in the child and is potentially harmful to his future personality development and emotional stability. These studies show that parents suffer too. Because they are rendered powerless to help the child, their confidence in themselves as parents is diminished. They may be affected in ways that may have a profound influence on the future mental health of the family.

As these effects have come to be better understood, attempts have been made to make the hospital a happier place for children. Visiting hours for parents have been extended, and a few hospitals even provide facilities for parents to stay overnight. Playrooms and a variety of toys are provided. Bright colors and murals may be used to make the surroundings more cheerful. The child may be dressed in gay hospital clothing, and the nurses may wear colorful dresses rather than white uniforms.

These changes have undoubtedly been helpful, especially for older children. But they do not meet the needs of the preschool child, whose primary need is for close and continuous contact with his mother. Neither do they meet the needs of the parents.

A further and crucial change is necessary. We need to revise our thinking so that we do not focus almost exclusively on the needs of the child. It may be that at any given moment the parent needs help from the nurse more than the child does. The parent's need cannot be isolated from the child's need. The emotional ties between parent and child are too strong to allow for fragmentation of care. We are faced with the challenge of providing maternal-child nursing, or "parent-child nursing" as it is sometimes more appropriately called.

To understand the need for taking this step, consider what happens to the child when he enters the hospital and is separated from his mother. A common pattern of behavior may be observed. First is a period of *protest*, usually lasting about three days, during which the child makes frantic efforts to bring the lost object (mother) back. He cries loudly and expresses his anger violently. He clings to a favorite toy or object from home and will not allow it to be taken from him. He resists the efforts of nurses to give physical care, and responds with hostility. When mother or father visits, he cries and clings to the parent. When the parent leaves, he screams and cries and cannot be consoled.

About the fourth day the child gives way to *despair*. His efforts to retrieve the lost object have failed, and the adaptive value of continued resistance fades because of his need for physical care and protection. He now accepts physical care with less protest and may seem to have adjusted to the new situation. At this time nurses are apt to say that the child has "gotten used to the hospital." He responds more readily to the efforts of new adults to divert him and to win a smile, but signs of regression can be observed: reduced use of words, lapse of sphincter control (apt to produce extreme anxiety), increase in biting and other aggressive behavior. When the parents visit, the child may almost ignore the mother and turn instead to the father.

This phase may be followed by a period of *detachment*, when there is a loosening of ties to the parents. The child may seldom cry for the parents now, and may forget or ignore the favorite object or toy from home. When the parents visit, he shows delight; but this is directed more to the gifts they have brought than to the parents. It is as though he has lost faith in the parents as a source of gratification and turns instead to oral gratification and possession of material objects. Such a reaction is ominous for his future emotional health and personality development, and for his ability to form warm and rewarding relationships.

The intensity of harmful effects varies with the age of the child. The infant under age 1 suffers less than the toddler because he responds more readily to substitute mothers. The 4- to 6-year-old may respond in ways similar to those of the younger child, but he is able to adapt himself more readily, is better able to understand and accept time concepts and explanations, and is capable of more postponement of wish-fulfillment. It is the 1-to 3-year-old who is most vulnerable to the effects of separation.

Many parents now recognize that separation during hospitalization causes suffering and regression in children, and they hesitate to submit a child to hospitalization because they fear this experience may cause greater damage than the disease. Most doctors do not recommend hospitalization if it can be avoided.

Often, parents complain that nurses are restrictive and authoritarian, and fail to see the child's need for his parents and the parents' need to be with the child. They say nurses may tell them they cannot stay with the child because it is against hospital rules when, in fact, such rules do not exist. They complain that nurses do not want information the parents are eager to give about the child, but treat them as though the nurses knew the child better than the parents do.

It seems strange that parents have not banded together and insisted on their right to remain with sick children, as they have insisted on "rights" in other areas (for example, the right of the father to be present in the delivery room). However, a sick child in need of hospitalization precipitates a crisis and the parents may be unable to function normally. Their first reaction is denial and disbelief, followed by fear and frustration that is often coupled with depression and guilt. The upset, grieving, possibly guilt-ridden parents are in no position to demand their "rights," particularly when they fear that further insistence may prejudice the child's treatment. However, it is possible that if changes in child care are not made soon, parents *will* band together and demand to participate in giving care. If this happens, nurses will lose much of the leadership role that would enable them to be truly helpful to children and parents.

As for the nurse, her emotional involvement in caring for children may also be frustrating. With the highest of motives she assumes the mother-surrogate role and strives to meet the needs of the hospitalized child. With equally high motives she endeavors to protect both parent and child by being a buffer between them. She may not realize that she is protecting herself too by avoiding the need to cope with both parent and child simultaneously. She was not taught to work *with* parents in caring for sick children or in planning for their care after discharge. No one has helped her to see that the maintenance of the parent-child relationship has a higher priority than the smooth running of the hospital ward.

There have always been compassionate and understanding nurses who have been as helpful to parents as they could possibly be under the prevailing system. Many a weary mother has been given coffee and a warm blanket by the nurse as the mother sat through a long night beside her sick child. Many an anxious father has found his way up the back stairs, knowing that the nurse would permit him to spend a few minutes with his child even though he could not visit during hours. Many a nurse has been torn between enforcing hospital policy and giving way to her feeling that parents and children need each other. The tragedy is that all too often nurses do not take the initiative to see that policies which violate modern concepts of patient care are changed.

There is an urgent need today for a realistic appraisal of nursing practices. Persons involved in caring for sick children within a given institution should agree on the philosophy and goals that determine the priority to be given to the various aspects of care. They should ask themselves: What is most important in caring for children? Which practices are helpful to children and parents, and which are harmful? How can we minimize the harmful effects of hospitalization? How can we strengthen the parent-child relationships?

Once these questions are answered, changes in practice can be introduced gradually and given a fair chance and an honest evaluation. But first all personnel should be convinced of the need for changes and committed to the philosophy on which the changes are based. This can be accomplished with a good inservice education program in which all are involved and the contributions of all are valued.

An educational program is needed to help the nurses increase their understanding of the needs of children and parents, and also their understanding of their own motivations, reactions, and needs. Resource persons available in the wider community can be helpful in this program. Also, nurses need to be given the opportunity to take college courses and to attend pertinent workshops, conferences, and professional meetings. Ideally, a maternal and child health nurse-specialist should be added to the staff to provide wise and expert supervision and serve as a role model.

After the desired changes have been instituted, what should the nurse's role be in a parent-child nursing program?

First, she promotes the mental health of parents and child not only by permitting the parents to be with the child in the hospital and participate in his care but by *encouraging* them to do so. She helps make this experience as comfortable and rewarding as possible. If a mother has difficulty deciding where her first responsibility lies, the nurse helps her look at the family situation and arrive at a solution that best meets the needs of the total family. If the mother cannot stay with the sick child, the nurse helps the parents understand the meaning of the child's subsequent behavior and the ways in which they can minimize the effects of separation.

She also helps the parents understand the reasons for behavioral changes they will see when the child returns home, and she makes suggestions for dealing with them. She may explain, for example, that the child's sense of trust and his sense of autonomy have been violated by this experience. He may show lack of affection toward the mother and resist her attempts to feed and dress him. If the parents respond with counter-aggression, there is little hope of restoring a strong parent-child relationship. Time, understanding, and careful nurturing are necessary.

She may explain, further, how important play is to children, both in the hospital and at home. The young child expresses feelings in play that he cannot express in words. Thus parents (and nurses) need to be able to tolerate a good deal of play activity and hostility. When a child is allowed freedom of expression through this channel, he can begin to master his fears and gain release from tension and aggressive feelings.

"The very first requirement of a hospital," wrote Florence Nightingale in her "Notes on Hospitals," "is that it should do the sick no harm."

Surely those words are as pertinent today as yesterday! It is time to take a fresh look at the care of young children in the hospital. It is time to replace child-centered nursing with parent-child nursing.

What signs of regression can be observed in a preschool-age child? What periods precede the period of regression? What follows it?

How can a nurse adapt to restrictive hospital policies and still support the relationships between children and parents?

Why must nurses accept this responsibility?

How can you find out what the philosophy is in the children's unit in your community?

How could you go about promoting change if you feel it is necessary? How can attitudes be changed so that actual nursing practice can change?

Reread this article at the end of your nursing program and list some positive steps you can take to promote parent-child nursing.

How are the nurse's communication skills used here? How and why does a nurse encourage parents to make decisions? How does she prepare the parents for the convalescent period?

PART IV

SOME BASIC SKILLS

What are the basic skills of nursing? The lists are long and varied, limited only by the people giving nursing care to those individuals needing care. In this group you will find selections on situations that commonly occur. Many of these may not be on your "skills list," but a skilled nurse would be skilled in all of these. Think about it!

The term "skills" is used for Parts IV and V to imply that nursing care, procedures, and techniques, for example, are indeed skills to be learned, practiced, improved, and changed as nurses become more experienced. Observing patients for fluids and electrolytes imbalance is just as much a skill as giving an injection. We must broaden our viewpoint of what we traditionally think of as nursing skills.

For those of you who are new to nursing, Part IV will give you an overview of what varied knowledge and skills are required of a nurse. If you are an R.N., these articles will both reinforce and help you recall what basics of nursing care you learned many years ago, as well as introducing you to some of the newer points of view that are enlarged upon in later articles.

PREPARING

31.
Preparing Children for Procedures and Operations

Mary Scahill

Growth and development is the key to relating to children. You must know what to expect at each stage of growth in order to best help a child adjust to a hospital stay. You must not expect to be able to remember all the details of each stage. Review what is expected of each age group in a growth and development reference as you prepare to care for patients from 1 to 18 years of age.

The nurse who would help the pediatric patient withstand the emotional and physical trauma that may accompany a particular procedure, surgical or otherwise, must keep in mind that within the body being treated there lives a child. If he is accorded respect and dignity, if he is dealt with in a sincere and kindly manner, if he is told the truth and given encouragement, then he can be expected to achieve some degree of self-mastery and ego growth no matter how difficult his situation. In order to help the child, those caring for him must understand their own feelings. The nurse who is faced with a difficult task—changing a burn dressing, for example, which often creates an unimagined amount of pain—may be deeply troubled by her feelings of helplessness and anxiety. The surgeon who must amputate a child's leg may suffer untold emotional agony. Staff conferences in which personnel feel free to verbalize their feelings enable the various members to give support to each other as they recognize in each other some of their own needs. Thus, the nurse who has to do a painful dressing can discuss the procedure in a conference and everyone who deals with the child will know what is going to happen. When the child cries they will know that his pain is very real and that the nurse is well aware of it. As a result, when the child talks about the incident later—in the playroom, for instance—other workers are prepared to let him verbalize his feelings and to help him understand why the procedure was necessary, thereby helping him rebuild his trust account which was drawn upon during the painful experience. If we expect the child to trust us, we must trust the child by giving to him and remaining sensitive to his needs even when he does not respond.

EVERYTHING IS STRANGE

When the child is admitted to the hospital, he enters a strange environment and is immediately surrounded by strange people, equipment, and noises. We should strive to keep the amount of strangeness to a minimum. The parents can assist and support us as we introduce him to the ward, show him where the bathroom is, where the playroom is, where he can get a drink of water, and what is in his bedside stand. He needs to be told how he can call the nurse, the head nurse's name and, most important of all, his own nurse's name. Large and fearful equipment should be kept out of sight. Any special rules should be explained to him so that he may feel free to exercise his independence without getting into trouble. Not too many people should be involved in his care, at least not until he has had time to adjust to some of the strangeness. His parents should be helped to leave if they cannot stay, and the nurse should make sure that they tell him they are leaving and when they expect to return.

During the first few days following his admission to the hospital, the ground work is laid for his responses to procedures that may need to be carried out later, including surgery should that be necessary.

With ego support as a goal, we can help the child cope with the reality of his situation by meeting his dependency needs and assisting him toward independence. Therefore, if we tell him what to expect and how he may help, we were capitalizing on his inner strengths. A friendly approach with time for him to ask questions is one way to achieve success. Let him help with a dressing by tearing off a wrapper or holding a bandage in place while you tape it. If possible, allow him to select the injection site and help scrub the area.

Jimmy was a 10-year-old who required wet dressings several times a day. The nurse took him into the treatment room where privacy was assured and he could feel free to cry out if necessary without embarrassment. She had him put on a mask and sterile gloves. As he removed the old dressing, she told him to let her know when to soak it more to alleviate discomfort. She told him how the wound was healing and, as she applied the new wet bandages, asked him to hold them in place while she wrapped the leg. Jimmy felt very proud of his accomplishment. Thus, she created a feeling of mutual trust, and he achieved control over his body.

The hospitalized infant needs to be provided with some way of dealing with his anxiety. A pacifier or a bottle will give him some satisfaction. Up to the age of four, a child does not understand why the hurt is necessary and he needs comfort and support. This may be provided by the presence of a calm nurse—or similar person—who talks to him in soft tones, fondles and strokes him gently, or diverts his attention temporarily with a toy or by singing a familiar song.

Some children may pretend a bravado which is artificial. Boys of school age often think it sissyish to admit that something hurts. Because our culture assigns a priority to boys being brave and strong, a boy in the hospital feels he must still be brave. The staff members should assure him that to admit to pain and to being afraid is no reflection on his personal integrity and character. It's quite all right to say it hurts; and to yell when it does.

An operation is very frightening to a child, particularly when he is unprepared for it. Consider for a moment what the child must endure—strange surroundings, strange people dressed in unfamiliar looking clothes, frightening equipment, other children who cry out in pain, a tremendous amount of activity that revolves around him, plus anxious parents who seem powerless to reassure him. Certainly, he thinks, something dreadful is about to happen. He is told to lie still, not to throw things and, most of all, to be quiet and to be a "good boy." Overwhelmed by terror, he must be passive. He wakens from anesthesia, feels sick, and is in pain. One arm or leg may be tied down and the other may have a long tube stuck into it that comes from a bottle turned upside down hanging from a funny looking pole. The bottle may even be filled with blood and this increases his anxiety. In addition, he is in a different room from the one he occupied preoperatively, and strange people dressed in blue—or maybe green—keep coming in to check on him: they take his blood pressure and his pulse, or they stick a thermometer into his rectum—all the while speaking in hushed voices with or without explanation. His parents are nowhere to be seen and he is certain they will never find him.

Not knowing what has happened, the young patient's imagination conjures up fantastic ideas that increase his terror if no attempt is made to correct them. . . .The fantasies he develops lead him to deal with the situation either by attacking the cause, which is the doctor, or by running away and withdrawing into himself.

PREPARATION IS ALL-IMPORTANT

Many of the child's fears and anxieties can be alleviated by adequate preparation prior to surgery. Such preparation should start before he enters the hospital. It needs to be done gradually by someone he trusts, beginning with the parents and the doctor. After admission, he needs to have opportunities to talk about his conceptions of the operation, and of what is going to be done and why. The explanation of his particular operation should be repeated several times before the surgery is performed, and his questions and ideas elicited. Children who are eight or more years of age may be shown a simple outline of the body with the affected area indicated. The adolescent will benefit from a more lifelike anatomical drawing or model and may want a detailed account of how the particular body part functions. On the other hand, some adolescents become threatened by too much information, and will tolerate only a general description. For young children, unable to comprehend what they do not see, a simple explanation that the doctor is going to fix something inside that is making him sick is adequate and will reassure him.

The child should know whether or not he will have a dressing, a cast, or some other special appliance. To wake up in a body cast or in traction with ropes running every which way stimulates all kinds of additional anxieties. The child who has had his head shaved is afraid to ask what has happened. A girl, in particular, feels mutilated. She should know that her hair will grow in again and that there are all kinds of pretty scarfs and hats that she may wear in the interim to make her look no different than her friends.

ONE CHILD'S RESPONSE

The following incident illustrates one child's preparation for and response to surgery.

Timmy, aged six, two days after plastic surgery on his ears, wore a complete head dressing with only his face exposed. He was a handsome lad with bright blue eyes and a sunny smile. I asked him if he knew what type of operation he had had. He replied, "the doctor fixed my ears." When I asked him if the doctor had told him what his bandage would be like, he answered, "Yes, and he told me I musn't lie on this ear," pointing to the affected ear. I said, "Do you know what the bandage looks like?" Timmy answered that he did not. I offered to hold him up in front of the mirror which was too high for him to see in by himself. He climbed into my arms and was so happy to see that he really did look like he was wearing a space helmet.

Timmy was quite at ease with himself because he had been told exactly what to expect. He did not lie on the affected ear and was able to talk about his experience.

The child who must undergo surgery and face anesthesia without preparation for it may be filled with terror. He is afraid that if he is put to sleep he may not wake up; he fears losing control over his body and of what might be done to it while he is asleep. A simple, truthful explanation that the reason for anesthesia is to spare him pain will comfort him. . . .If he does not know that the sleep will be induced gradually he may think he is dying. The younger child cannot comprehend all of the details but, if he has the experience of having the mask put on his face in play before coming to the hospital, he will be less afraid. Children of all ages will benefit from this type of practice. A visit by the anesthetist and the recovery room nurse before surgery will also do much to make his postoperative adjustment easier.

COMMUNICATION IS THE KEY

If the parents are the best persons to assume the responsibility for preparing their child for procedures and operations, why do they often fail to do so? Much of the blame rests with the professional personnel. Medical care has become so highly specialized and hospital care so complicated that the end result is often an impersonal and routinized regimen. Who bothers to tell the parents about the countless x-rays in darkened rooms, the endless stream of specialists who must each examine the child, the many blood tests and other diagnostic measures that must be taken?

How can we help parents help their child cope with the stresses of procedures and operations? The most important way is to open the avenues of communication. Even the busy doctor can take time to inform the child of expected treatments and changes. The nurse can take time to explain and clarify ongoing and future events. She can share with the parents the details of the child's progress or lack of it; how well or how poorly he is eating; why he behaves as he does; and what type of play he engages in while they are absent. She can urge and encourage the parents to participate in the child's care, thereby providing them with a natural means of continuing the parent-child contact inherent in their reciprocal roles.

One cardiac-unit nurse visited at home the family of a child who was to have heart surgery so that she could learn about the family interactions, become familiar with the parents and child, and explain some of the things that would happen in the hospital. She brought along a doll with a catheter and an intravenous needle inserted, and the incision site marked. She also brought a book with pictures of some of the equipment. She discussed hospital routines and ways in which the parents could help the child develop positive attitudes toward the doctors and nurses. Because of the several home visits she made before the child was admitted, hers was a familiar face to them when they arrived at the hospital, and they leaned on her for support. The parents developed a trust in the nurse and the hospital and were able to impart this attitude to their child.

Involvement of the total family can be fostered through encouraging the parents to discuss with the children who are left at home what is going on in the hospital. They may need the nurse's assistance in planning how to explain the situation and what words they should use. In this way, the integrity of the family is both maintained and strengthened.

After he has experienced a painful procedure, the child should be provided with a means of working off his anger in words and aggressive play. Otherwise the anger lingers on. He sees the experience as an expression of hostility and wants to retaliate. One such activity is situational doll play with real hospital equipment. This relieves some of the tension and assists him to assimilate the reality. Although the procedure may hurt just as much the next time, he will have had an opportunity to familiarize himself with all of its various trappings. His pride will have been bolstered and his ego reinforced.

SUMMARY

Children have the ability to face and endure pain if they are adequately prepared for it. The nurse who recognizes her own feelings about hurting children and deals with them in a positive manner is better equipped to help the child deal with his. By discussing the child's fantasies and feelings with him, the nurse can help him achieve some mastery over himself. By involving parents as much as possible the nurse helps them, too, to cope with their feelings and, in addition, contributes to the maintenance of the integrity of the family unit.

List your expectations of Jimmy and Timmy because of their age. How would you change your preparation and teaching if Jimmy were three and Timmy 15. Why?

Should a physician, nurse, or parent do the preparation and teaching for a child? How do you find out? What is the nurse's role in each instance?

32.
Group Instruction in Preparation for Surgery

Elizabeth Jane Mezzanotte

Groups are another way to help patients prepare for surgery. Compare the purpose and results of group teaching with that of teaching individual patients as you read the following article.

Adequate preoperative instruction of patients has been credited with decreasing patient anxiety, decreasing postoperative vomiting, allaying fear about postoperative pain, and increasing, postoperative activity. However, because this instruction is given individually and, therefore, takes a considerable amount of time, some surgical patients still receive only a minimum amount of instruction.

Why not, then, instruct several preoperative patients at the same time? Group instruction incorporates such advantages as more adequate instruction for more patients, a definite time and place for the instruction, a consistent presentation of the instructions, and designation of one nurse to give the instruction, Moreover, it offers the patient the potentially therapeutic value of participation in a group.

The theory of group learning states that through participation in groups, a person is apparently stimulated to meet goals beyond those he would conquer as an isolate. Individuals also have a tendency to identify with others having similar goals or problems, and they gain moral support and encouragement through this identification. Group learning is also enhanced by the interaction among group members.

Group instruction sessions have been used extensively in such areas of health education as prenatal care, postpartum and infant care, child care, and diabetes, to name a few. The attractiveness of group learning in health education is evidenced by the numbers of persons who assemble with others having similar health problems to receive instruction and exchange ideas, as in colostomy clubs, larnygectomee clubs, and so on.

The study was limited to patients having elective abdominal surgery. Six groups of patients, averaging four patients per group, were given detailed preoperative instructions that followed a planned outline, including four major areas of information: (1) general instructions in preparation for surgery, (2) hospital policies concerning surgical patients, (3) suggestions about the control of pain, (4) activity that would promote satisfactory recovery. Patients were encouraged to ask questions and participate in the discussion. Classes were held at 6:00 P.M. the day prior to surgery and lasted approximately 30 minutes. The time was selected because it followed the supper hour and did not interfere with the patient's visitors. No attempt was made to discuss specific care that would require medical orders.

One 83-year-old woman was hesitant about attending the session because she said that she was so forgetful. With encouragement, however, she decided to attend.

Once in the group session, some patients contributed information from their own observations. One suggested that taking a few deep breaths at night before going to sleep helped him to relax. Another patient expressed definite goals: "I'm glad to know about the exercises. I want to get up the day of surgery and go home by the seventh day."

One patient expressed relief: "I'm glad that it's O.K. to move around in bed and be able to lie on your side."

Some were philosophic: "When you come to the hospital and you think so many people are well, you feel sorry for yourself. When you get here and see how big the hospital is and how many people are sick, you know you're not so bad off, at that."

Another patient commented, "When you meet with other people having surgery too, you don't feel so alone."

One patient remarked apprehensively, "Tomorrow we won't be feeling so well."

Exercises were explained and practiced during the session and, for reinforcement, an instruction sheet describing them was distributed.

During the instruction, some patients responded with, "That's good to know," or "That I knew." All patients showed a definite interest in the instruction. Their questions included the following:

"Can I go to communion in the morning?" "Can I go to mass in the chapel tomorrow?" "Does everyone have gas pains?" "If your heart stops during

PATIENT INSTRUCTION SHEET
FOR A BETTER RECOVERY AFTER YOUR SURGERY

Repeat the following exercise every 1-2 hours until you are up and around.
Nurses will assist you if you have any difficulty or any questions.

KEEP LUNGS FUNCTIONING PROPERLY! ! !

DEEP
BREATHE
AND
COUGH! ! !

1. Inhale as deeply as you can.
2. Hold for a second or two.
3. Exhale completely.
4. Repeat several times. Then:
5. Inhale deeply.
6. Produce a deep abdominal cough (not shallow throat cough) by short, sharp expiration. (Incision may be splinted with hands or bedclothes. Flexing knees relieves strain on abdominal muscles.)

MAINTAIN GOOD CIRCULATION! ! !
Lie on each side as well as on your back.

CHANGE
POSITION! ! !

To turn easily:
1. Determine the direction of your turn.
2. Lift that arm overhead.
3. Bend the opposite knee, planting your foot firmly on the bed.
4. Pushing with bent leg, roll onto your side (bedrails can be used to aid in turning).
5. If you need assistance, call one of the nurses.

To turn back again:
1. Bend knee of upper leg.
2. Place palm of top arm solidly on the side of the bed.
3. Push yourself over onto your back.

PROMOTE GOOD CIRCULATION IN YOUR LEGS! ! !

EXERCISE
FEET
AND
LEGS! ! !

Perform the following exercises *fairly slowly,* but with strong muscle contraction.

1. Push the toes of both feet toward the foot of the bed. Relax both feet. Pull toes toward the chin. Relax both feet.
2. Circle both ankles, first to the right; then to the left. Repeat three times. Relax.
3. Bend each knee alternately, sliding foot up along the bed. Relax.

surgery, would the doctor open your chest to get it started again?" "Is it all right to cough after you have a hernia operation?" "Will I be getting out of bed on the day of my operation?" "How soon will I get up after surgery?" "Will I have to remove my false teeth when I go to the operating room?" "Can I leave my wedding ring on?"

A 75-year-old woman commented that at first she had thought she was too old to have surgery. One of the other patients in the group answered her, saying, "My mother was 77 when she fell and broke her hip. She came out of the surgery just fine."

Following the session, the patients were escorted back to their rooms. Comments made and questions asked by patients during the session were later recorded, and pertinent information was incorporated into the plan of instruction for succeeding group sessions.

RESULTS

The most frequent comment—by 15 patients—was that they had gained the ability to participate properly in the activity after surgery. Twelve patients said they received answers to their questions; 12 said they learned how to improve their recovery; 11 said they liked meeting with other patients scheduled for surgery; 7 reported liking the group discussion; and 2 said the session lessened their anxiety.

Their specific comments included the following: "Other people suggest things that you don't think of." "There's emphasis on the important things." "Knowing what to expect was helpful." "You don't feel you're the only one having an operation. Others are in the same boat." "I got rid of phlegm by deep breathing and coughing and holding my incision." "Exercising helped me get up sooner." "Deep breathing helped me get rid of the bad taste."

One patient commented that when he woke up after surgery he could not move or talk, but he thought of the deep breathing, he did it, and it seemed to help him.

When asked to state a preference for either the group instruction or a shorter period of individual instruction, 20 said they preferred the group session, one was uncertain, and two said that they would prefer individual instruction. One man said that with the individual instruction, "You could ask more questions and not feel backward."

The 83-year-old woman said the individual instruction might be better for her because she was forgetful. However, her daughter, who was in the room during the interview, reported that when her mother returned from the recovery room, she said, "I have to take deep breaths and I have to move my legs." So she did seem to have remembered something of her preoperative instruction.

All 23 patients said that if a relative or friend were to have surgery, they would recommend the group instruction.

In retrospect, the plan of instruction seemed adequate and could be presented comfortably in 30 minutes. To give comparable instruction to an equal number of surgical patients individually would require that many times the 30 minutes needed for a group session. In addition, patients instructed individually would be deprived of the benefits they gained from meeting with the group. It would appear, though, that some surgical patients would profit most from a combination of group and individual instruction.

Naturally, should a plan of group instruction in preparation for surgery be adopted, an individual nurse's responsibility for giving instruction and psychologic support to surgical patients would not cease with the patients' attendance at the group sessions. As one patient noted, some persons have questions that they would not ask because they are in a group.

However, if preoperative instructions had been given to the group, the nurse could spend more time with those patients who do have special problems or who need specific attention, reassured that she has not neglected the needs of the many for the few.

List some advantages of group instruction as compared with individual patient instruction and give reasons for each choice.

What four areas of instruction were covered for each patient group in this study? How do you cover each of these areas when preparing patients for surgery?

How do you think unique, physical, and mental problems for a particular patient could be handled?

After reading article #46 "Three Days with Mrs. M." review the patient comments in this article and list cues from these comments that might indicate a problem that you would want to pursue on a one-to-one basis.

How does this group differ from the one described in selection #6 "Handicapped Patients Talk Together"?

Which group would you prefer to organize and lead and why?

33.

Confusion in the Management of Diabetes

Julia D. Watkins
Fay T. Moss

Patients with chronic disease, perhaps more than many other people, must know the reason for each treatment or action in order to prevent complications. This kind of situation gives you a wealth of opportunity to teach the reasons and to evaluate the patient's learning. As you read this article, list or underline all of the items to be taught (and learned). In this instance, before reading why and how each item is taught, write how you would teach it and why.

Because so many persons with diabetes appear healthy and carry on normal work and social activities, it is perhaps easy to forget that the diabetic patient's condition, as much as any other chronic state, affects and is affected by the basic needs of life—food, activity, relationship with others—every hour of the day.

The patient is expected to remember and to administer medication accurately at least once and sometimes several times a day, to make frequent tests of urine specimens, and to consider the consequence of every bit of food he eats as well as to balance his food and medication with his activity. Ordinary indiscretions in eating and the human characteristics of forgetfulness and error-making, which might not be serious in other situations, for the diabetic may make the difference between being admitted to or staying out of the hospital, or even between life and death.

INSULIN ADMINISTRATION

In our experience, a major source of patients' confusion is the variety of syringes and insulins available. Another is the sterilization process.

While there is a large variety of insulin syringes available, three basic types are generally used: the single scale U-40, the single scale U-80 (short and long types), and the dual scale U-40–80. These are available as reusable glass syringes and disposable plastic syringes, with the exception of the long U-80 syringe which is available only in glass. Calibrations on both the glass and plastic U-40 syringe are in one-unit increments. On the short-type glass and on the plastic U-80 syringe, calibrations are in two-unit increments, and on the long-type glass U-80 they are in one-unit increments. On the U-40–80 syringe, the same markings indicate one unit on the U-40 side and two units on the U-80 side.

Patients who are taught in the hospital or doctor's office to measure insulin in one type of syringe may easily purchase another to use at home and therefore make serious dosage errors. For example, during his hospitalization Mr. H. was taught to withdraw insulin to "four marks above the 20 line" on a glass U-80 syringe, long type. Upon discharge, he was given a supply of disposable U-80 syringes. He continued to measure to four marks above the 20 line and was, therefore, taking 28, not 24 units of insulin.

Another possible source of error involves the incorrect matching of syringes and insulins. A patient may measure one strength of insulin in a syringe that is calibrated for another strength. For example, both Mrs. T. and her doctor stated that she took 20 units of insulin, but she was measuring U-80 insulin in a U-40 syringe, and was actually getting 40 units.

Also, the patient may attempt to rely only on the color of the syringe and the insulin cap in determining which insulin to take, since syringes are marked in red for the U-40 strength and green for the U-80 strength. However, patients may use the wrong type of insulin if they believe that it is sufficient to match a red syringe with a red insulin bottle, because all vials of U-40 insulin—long, intermediate, and short-acting—are marked with red, and all types of U-80 insulin are marked with green.

The dual U-40–80 syringe is still in use and may cause dual problems. That is, the patient may use the set of calibrations which does not match his insulin and measure either twice the prescribed dose, or one half the prescribed dose. Mr. B., a known diabetic of long standing, whose diabetes for many months had been under fairly good control, was admitted to the hospital with acute and severe hypoglycemia. Investigation by the public health nurse disclosed that for three days prior to hospitalization he had received a double dose of insulin. The daughter who usually had measured the dose became "tired" of doing so and had given the responsibility to her sister, who measured it on the wrong side of the U-40–80 syringe.

It is important that the patient understands that various types of syringes are available, and that he learns to choose the one to which he is accustomed. Miss E., a new diabetic, learned how to administer her insulin in a single scale U-40 syringe. Upon discharge she was given written instructions about the type of syringe to buy. But in her local drugstore, she was sold a dual scale syringe and told it would "do just as well."

One of the major misinterpretations about sterilization of syringes seems to involve a lack of understanding of why sterilization is necessary, Mr. R. stated that he had been taught to boil his syringe every time he used it. But he said he followed this instruction carefully by boiling the syringe *after* each injection and then storing it in a small cardboard box. Obviously, patients need to be taught why they should do something in terms that make the process have meaning for them.

Patients often think they can sterilize disposable syringes as they do glass ones, and reuse them. In fact, patients report that they are told to do so by health professionals. Since the cost of these syringes is a large item in the budget of many persons, they are often reluctant to throw them away after just one use. Soaking and boiling, as well as handling, cause the markings to become unclear and eventually to disappear entirely from plastic syringes.

URINE TESTING

Patients show confusion about which specimen is to be tested, how to use the prescribed test, and how to read the test.

So often one hears patients told to test an "early morning specimen." Does the patient know this should be the *second* specimen, voided within an hour of emptying the bladder the first time? Does the patient realize the specimen to be tested should be voided *before* taking insulin as well as before eating breakfast? Does the patient realize that specimens to be tested at other times of the day also should be second voided specimens?

There are a number of different urine sugar tests available. Patients seem to find out about them in various ways and may try them out, especially if they seem less costly or easier than the one they were taught to use. Each test must be carried out in its own specific way in order to produce an accurate reading. Details which may seem unimportant to patients may be overlooked; some steps may be omitted entirely from the procedure. For example, touching or wetting the "business" end of the stick tests may invalidate results. If waiting periods are not observed before reading the tests as indicated, results may be false, so the nurse should remember to emphasize the importance of these waiting periods and help the patient who may not have a watch or clock with a seocnd hand to devise a method for estimating the passing of time.

Continuous observation of the color changes is another point which may be overlooked. Mrs. C. read her test after an accurately determined waiting period but failed to observe the intermediate stages and therefore recorded a result which indicated a much lower sugar content than the test actually indicated.

The color chart accompanying each test is different. Patients who have used several tests may easily interchange these color charts and obtain incorrect readings. For example, whereas yellow for one test indicates no sugar content, with another test yellow indicates a fairly high percentage of sugar. Also, the code of 1+, 2+, and so forth, indicates a different sugar percentage on different tests.

Since the physician may base the prescribed insulin dose partly on urine test results, it is very important not only to know what the patient says his urine sugars are, but also to explore with him what specimen he used, what test he used, how he did the test, what color chart he read, and how he read it.

DIET

Confusion about diet seems to arise most frequently in converting a meal plan into day-to-day eating habits. Often after extensive review of a dietary regimen, the patient remembers only that he must eat no sugar and must use fat sparingly in cooking. Exchange lists seem particularly confusing to some patients.

Patients often have a written copy of their meal plan which has been carefully calculated to fit their insulin and exercise regimens. They can produce such a copy, carefully folded, from between pages of a book or from a drawer where it has been kept "so I wouldn't lose it." Further investigation may uncover two extremes, such as Mr. W., who shyly complained, "For the last 12 years I have eaten a slice of cheese, four crackers, and half a glass of milk before going to bed. I'm a little tired of cheese," and Mrs. S., who brushed off the nurse with, "My friend's doctor just told her to avoid sweets." Was translation of the plan into action too complicated, too confusing, or unrealistic?

Susie T. was faced with a dilemma: she had been told by the dietician how to plan each meal carefully according to the physician's prescription. She had also been told by the same physician to eat the regular lunch served at school.

Mrs. H. had her diet and insulin regimen carefully prescribed for daily meals at 8:00, 12:00, and 6:00. However, her husband worked on evening shifts, and this schedule of meals was not in keeping with her daily routine.

Mrs. E. was given a meal plan including meat twice a day when her children did not have shoes. Is it strange that many patients have the reaction expressed by one, "The doctors and nurses don't know how to help me; I have to treat myself as best I can"?

COMBATING CONFUSION

Newer knowledge brings changes in the treatment of diabetes. The invention of newer and "better" gadgets and techniques provides increased choices in management. Mobility of the population often means a patient faces frequent change in professional contacts. Keeping confusion for the patient at a minimum is a challenge. Keeping things simple can in itself be a confusing task. What can the nurse do to reduce unnecessary confusion?

First, she needs to get the facts. She must determine exactly what the patient *is doing* and exactly what the doctor *expects*. Conversations with the patient and/or family do not produce sufficient information. Whenever possible the nurse must gain her knowledge of what the patient is doing by careful observation and skillful interviewing, because patients have often learned the "right" answers to the questions which they are repeatedly asked—answers which may bear little resemblance to their performance of self-care. The nurse needs to know what the doctor means by his prescribed regimen. For example, when he writes, "1,800 cal. diabetic diet," how strict must this be? What spacing of feedings does he want?

Second, she should recognize her responsibility as go-between for physician and patient, so that she assists both of them in arriving at a mutually acceptable regimen which is clearly and realistically planned and stated.

Third, she needs to determine the patient's ability to learn, and then teach him in accordance with that ability. Much of the literature intended for patients and their families is written in language that requires a fairly high reading level and a middle-class frame of reference.

Fourth, the nurse should keep her own knowledge up to date. She should be familiar with the newer concepts of medical care and with the array of equipment and medications available.

Fifth, she needs to teach the patient safeguards he may use to avoid confusion, such as taking a broken syringe to the drugstore when buying a new one so that he will be certain to get another just like it, or asking the doctor for a written regimen when moving so the next doctor may have firsthand information immediately.

And, finally, the nurse should make periodic reassessments of the patient's management in order to ascertain the need for further clarification. Too often, once the patient has "learned" the techniques of care, the nurse has rejoiced in the independence of her patient and considered her job ended. However, as time passes, physiologic changes occur. The patient may also change his pattern of living, his marital status, his dwelling place, his job, his source of medical care.

We can never assume that a patient is performing as he was "taught." We must periodically determine whether he "learned" what we "taught," and whether what was taught is relevant to his present situation. For example, he may have learned to read his syringe correctly, but now he may be unable to see clearly.

Why is it essential that you have many samples of syringes when teaching about self-administration of insulin? Why must family members be involved in this learning? What problems might occur when converting a patient to U-100 insulin?

Why might role playing purchasing, and being responsible for their own insulin administration be helpful for patients in preparation for being discharged? You play the part of a pharmacist, a community health nurse or aide, an office nurse (telephone conversation), a family member, and a friend — use this technique for evaluating your patient's knowledge of the reason and the *importance* of rules learned from *your* teaching. Use the examples in this article to begin role playing.

List in short terms the six ways this article suggests for the nurse to reduce confusion to a diabetic patient. Keep this list handy and refer to it often. How would you evaluate how much understanding a patient has in each of these areas before beginning your teaching? How could you write this up as a nursing procedure?

OBSERVING

34.
Recognition, Significance, and Recording of the Signs of Increased Intracranial Pressure

Jessie F. Young

This is observation on a very high level. How do you know what to look for when the head and/or brain is injured? What signs and symptoms are ominous? Which are reportable? How do you describe them? How can you recognize change?

A METHOD OF TESTING AND RECORDING OBSERVATIONS OF NEUROSURGICAL PATIENTS

A method of testing and recording observations has been developed at the Toronto General Hospital, and is used routinely in evaluating neurosurgical patients. This method consists of assessing the patient's clinical state when he first comes under observation, and comparing his subsequent condition with the first record in order to detect changes that warn of an increase in intracranial pressure (Figure 1).

Case History 1

A construction laborer, aged 32, slipped on wet tiles, struck his head, and was rendered unconscious. After emergency treatment he was admitted to the intensive care area of the neurosurgical unit with a diagnosis of right temporal fracture and brain injury. He was placed on cranio-cerebral testing, a record of which is shown in Figure 2. On admission, he was drowsy, orientated to name only, and obeyed simple commands. The record demonstrated a gradual deterioration of consciousness. Two hours after admission to the unit he was semi-comatose, responding only to moderately painful stimuli. His right pupil reacted slowly to light, while the left continued to react briskly. Both arms and legs moved in response to moderatley painful stimuli, but the movements of the left side were weaker than those on the right. Blood pressure rose and pulse rate fell. An hour later, the patient was responding only to the most painful stimuli by movement of the right arm and leg and only slight movement in the left. The right pupil was now more dilated, though still reacting slowly. The record shows the changes from the time of admission to the unit at 1330 hours and over the next three hours, when the patient was taken to the operating room and a large right-sided extradural hematoma was removed.

This record demonstrates typical changes that occur with increasing intra-cranial pressure, caused in this instance by an extradural hematoma. It is important to begin treatment as soon as possible *before* such grave signs as pupillary fixation and spastic hemiplegia develop, and so the nurse observing the patient must *constantly compare* present findings with previous ones. The frequency of cranio-cerebral testing is ordered by the doctor. It varies from hourly to every four hours. In the event that an abnormal symptom arises, the testing should be repeated more frequently whether ordered or not. For example, when a patient who is on four-hourly testing becomes difficult to rouse and shows a rise in blood pressure, the frequency of testing of the abnormal symptoms should be increased to hourly or half-hourly.

Both the patient and the family should realize that testing is done routinely. If they understand the reason for these frequent interruptions they are reassured; if they do not, it is natural that they should suspect that intensive nursing activity signals a deterioration in the condition of the patient.

Change in a patient's condition may occur over a period of days, as in a patient with a chronic subdural hematoma, in a few hours, as in the above case of the laborer with an extradural hematoma, or in a matter of minutes, as shown in the following case.

Case History 2

A 24-year-old university student was involved in an automobile accident. On admission he was conscious and obeying commands. His main complaint was of severe, generalized headache. He was kept on very close cranio-cerebral testing overnight and his condition remained unchanged. In the morning he was alert, talking, and cooperative, but he still complained bitterly of a severe headache. During the day his condition remained unchanged. At 1730 hours he was reluctant to sit up and eat his supper. He was irritable and slightly drowsy. Ten minutes later an observant nurse found the patient could not be roused. On testing he was semi-comatose, responding only to deep pain. His blood pressure was 200/110 and pulse was 64; pupils were equal and reacted sluggishly to light. He was taken to the operating room at once where part of the frontal lobe, which was severely lacerated and swollen, was removed.

This case illustrates not only the swiftness of deterioration but also the subtlety of its early onset. Behavioral changes such as irritability, lethargy, failure to eat, and incontinence may precede the measurable signs outlined in the cranio-cerebral testing chart. Only through her own knowledge of the patient can the nurse detect these changes early. The head nurse and the surgeon should never minimize the nurse's observations.

THE USE OF THE CRANIO-CEREBRAL NURSING RECORD

The method of testing outlined in this article applies whether the patient is admitted to a small local hospital or to a large university teaching hospital. The necessary equipment for cranio-cerebral testing includes only a sphygmomano-meter, a stethoscope, a flashlight, and a watch. In a specialized unit the equipment may include electronic monitors and other mechanical devices.

Records should be neat, concise, and factual. They should provide pertinent information for the doctor. He is responsible for the diagnosis but his decision is frequently influenced by the nurse's observations. The nurse should record her observations following each cranio-cerebral testing, and must not be unduly influenced by the previous entry even though it is used for comparison. If a change has occurred rapidly her observations will differ markedly from the previous entry, and if in doubt she should not hesitate to have someone quickly verify her findings. Sudden changes should be underlined to assist the doctor when he is reviewing the record. To avoid repetition the notation "no change" is used if the testing observation is the same as the one previously recorded (Figure 2). At the end of each tour of duty fluid intake and output are totaled and the results transferred to the fluid balance sheet. The completed record is signed in case discussion or explanation may be required.

The sequence of the descriptive terms shown on the chart form in Figure 1 is based on the order of change as it occurs with increasing intracranial pressure. An explanation of each heading on the chart follows.

Level of Consciousness

A fall in the level of consciousness, whether or not accompanied by any noticeable change in the vital signs, is important and should be reported at once. *The state of consciousness is the single most important and most reliable index of the neurologic state.* The patient's state of consciousness is assigned to one of

TORONTO GENERAL HOSPITAL

NEUROSURGICAL
CRANIO-CEREBRAL NURSING RECORD

27457	1-6-69	
DUE	Jan. 6-69	1
	32	2
MR. JOHN		C
222 GREEN RD., TORONTO, ONT.		B
DR. J.T.		

DAY Monday   DATE Jan. 6   1969

ABBREVIATIONS
R3 – REACTING BRISKLY
R – REACTING
RS – REACTING SLOWLY
F – FIXED

HOUR	LEVEL OF CONSCIOUSNESS	B.P.	PULSE	PUPILS RIGHT	PUPILS LEFT	MOVEMENT & STRENGTH OF ARMS AND LEGS RIGHT (R)	LEFT (L)	TEMP.	RESP.	OTHER SYMPTOMS & OBSERVATIONS
	ALERT – Describe	Record each Reading	Record rate	Record –size –reaction to light		Compare right with left		Record each Reading	Record rate	For example
	e.g. – orientation					Record – equal or unequal				Abnormality of pulse, respiration, voiding, stools
	– ability to obey commands					Hand grasps – strong, weak, absent				Fluid leak: site, appearance, amount
	DROWSY – Describe					Arms and legs				
	e.g. – orientation					Movement – describe				Intravenous or blood: Reading and amount absorbed
	– ability to obey			RB • • RS		e.g. – spontaneous				
	– commands			R • • R		– to command				Drugs – only those ordered for a specific symptom
	STUPOROUS – Describe			RS • • RS		– to pain – light,				Special test – e.g. arteriogram
	e.g. response			RS ● • RB		moderate or deep.				Headache
	– to questioning			RB • ● RS						Vomiting
	– to light pain			F ● ●● F						Unusual behaviour
	– Ability to obey commands			F • • F						Speech disturbances
	SEMI-COMATOSE									Difficulty swallowing
	Responds only to pain – light, moderate or deep.									Seizure: Describe
	COMATOSE									Eyes: Ptosis, ocular deviation
	No response to deep pain									
	Any other observations									

Times as Ordered

FIGURE 1. Form for recording results of cranio-cerebral testing by the nurse, showing appropriate designations to be used.

228

TORONTO GENERAL HOSPITAL

NEUROSURGICAL
CRANIO-CEREBRAL NURSING RECORD

DAY __Monday__   DATE __Jan. 6__   1969

27457	1-6-69
DUE	Jan. 6-69
32	1
	2 C
	B

MR. JOHN
222 GREEN RD., TORONTO, ONT.
DR. J.T.

ABBREVIATIONS
RB – REACTING BRISKLY
R – REACTING
RS – REACTING SLOWLY
F – FIXED

HOUR	LEVEL OF CONSCIOUSNESS	B.P.	PULSE	PUPILS RIGHT	PUPILS LEFT	MOVEMENT & STRENGTH OF ARMS AND LEGS RIGHT (R)	LEFT (L)	TEMP.	RESP.	OTHER SYMPTOMS & OBSERVATIONS
1330	Drowsy – rouses easily.	110/70	74	RB	RB	Moves arms & legs spontaneously.		100	22	Haematoma – R.
	Orientated to name only.					Grasps firm and equal.				temporal – Seen by Dr. B.
	Obeys simple commands.									
1400	No change	115/70	74	RB	RB	No change		100	22	Emesis 100 c.c.
										Brownish fluid.
1445	Stuporous – responds only to	115/80	70	R	RB	Moves arms & legs to light pain.		100	22	Echogram done.
	light pain.					L. slower than R.				
1540	Semi-comatose – Responds to	130/80	68	RS	RB	Moves arms & legs to moderate pain.		100	24	Twitching – L. side of mouth.
	moderate pain.					L. slower and weaker than R.				Seen by Dr. B.
						TOTAL FLUID INTAKE 60 c.c. – sips of water				
						TOTAL FLUID OUTPUT Emesis 100 c.c.				
1615						Voided 350 c.c.				J. Jones
										500 c.c. Mannitol 20%
										I.V. started
1630	Semi-comatose – Responds only	136/80	70	RS	R	R. moves to	L. slight mov't.	101	18	Seen by Dr. B & Dr. T.
	to deep pain.					deep pain				
1645	Semi-comatose – Responds to	160/86	56	RS	R	R. moves slowly	L. slight mov't. –	101	16	Seen by Dr. T.
	repeated deep pain.					to deep pain.	weak.			
	Taken to Surgery									

FIGURE 2. Completed cranio-cerebral nursing record for one patient, covering three hours.

229

five levels—alert, drowsy, stuporous, semi-comatose, or comatose. The exact meaning of these terms, when used consistently, is understood by both the medical and the nursing staff working closely together. The term "unconscious" is not used, as it is too vague for accurate description. Some observations by which the level of consciousness is assessed are:

1. Orientation, as evaluated by conversational ability (in answer to questions as to person, place, and time).

2. *Ability to obey simple commands* such as, "Raise your right arm. Touch your left ear with your right hand."

3. *Response to painful stimuli* is used if the level of consciousness is stuporous or lower. The amount of painful stimulus required will of course vary with the patient's level of consciousness, and only the minimum stimulation needed to evoke a response should be applied. Record the patient's response to *light, moderate* or *deep* painful stimulation. These degrees of painful stimulation are gauged by the increasing amount and intensity of pressure applied and varies from minimal to severe. To test for pain, hold the patient's fingertip between your thumb and first finger. Apply pressure to the sides of the fingertip. (If the hands are covered and not accessible for testing, apply pressure to the Achilles tendon or to the tip of the little toe, using the same method as for the finger.) Do not use any method that leaves a mark or bruise, e.g., pinching the arm or chest; this is a sign of poor patient care. The type of response to pain is significant, for example purposeful resistance and withdrawal, as opposed to purposeless extensor spasm. The latter type of response signifies that the patient is functioning at a lower level of consciousness than the former.

Accurate evaluation rests on many factors other than those specifically mentioned here, and the experienced nurse knows that these must not be ignored. For example, ill patients admitted from another hospital, on being asked where they are, will usually name the hospital from which they were transferred. Answers may be delayed; patience and persistence are required. The nursing staff responsible for the patient's care over a sustained period is often more successful in eliciting verbal response than the neurosurgeon as he makes rounds.

Blood Pressure and Pulse Rate

A lowering in the level of consciousness due to increased intracranial pressure is usually followed by a *rise* in blood pressure and a *fall* in pulse rate. After surgery observations should be compared with those made during surgery and in the recovery room. The rise in blood pressure may be sudden or gradual, transitory or sustained. The clinical picture is distinct from cardiovascular shock in which the blood pressure falls and the pulse rate rises.

In measuring blood pressure the readings for the right arm may differ from those for the left. If there is such a difference the same arm should always be used so that a comparison can be made with the previous reading. If drugs are ordered, for example in the treatment of hypertension, this should be taken into consideration when evaluating the patient's condition. The characteristics of the pulse such as rhythm, regularity, and volume are recorded under "Other Symptoms and Observations."

Important as these observations are, it should be remembered that, as a rule, a rising blood pressure and a falling pulse are *later* signs of increasing intracranial pressure that develop *after* the level of consciousness has already begun to sink.

Pupillary Reaction

The method of recording the size and type of pupillary reaction is shown in Figures 1 and 2. First, compare and record the size and shape of the pupils. Second, using a flashlight, direct light into the eye under examination, while the other eye is covered. The pupil constricts if the reflex pathways have not been damaged. The presence or absence of response to light is most important. Normally, the pupil responds by a brisk constriction on exposure to light. This is recorded as "reacting briskly" (RB). In the early stages of oculomotor impairment of one eye due to the effects of raised intracranial pressure, the constriction is both less and slower than in the opposite eye. This is recorded as "reacting" (R). As the pressure continues to increase, the response becomes slower and is shown as "reacting slowly" (RS). Concurrently with the slowing down in reflex constriction the pupil increases in size. When oculomotor paralysis is advanced, the pupil fails to constrict when the retina is stimulated by light and is widely dilated. This is recorded as "fixed" (F).

Restless patients are frequently resistant to testing, and assistance may be required for proper evaluation. Pupillary reaction is a most important observation and if in doubt, the nurse must not hesitate to have her findings rechecked.

Movement and Strength of Arms and Legs

Observations of spontaneous movements should be made while giving routine care, for these are often as important as those made during craino-cerebral testing. Grasp of each hand is tested simultaneously for equality, strength of grasp, and ability to release. The movements of the arms and legs may be described as being spontaneous or in response to command. If the patient is moving to commands, describe the type of movement and any evidence of decreased motor power such as an inability to hold arms outstretched. A comparison is made between the right and left sides. If the patient is not obeying commands, then evaluate the movement of the arms and legs in response to painful stimuli, using the method already described. At the lowest level of consciousness the limbs assume a posture of extension and rigidity in response to deep painful stimulation.

Temperature

The temperature is taken rectally at specified times. The frequency of measurement should be increased if a marked change is noted. An electric or battery-operated thermometer with a rectal lead is used if temperatures are being taken frequently. With an elevation of temperature the possibility of infection should be considered; the common sites of infection are the chest, urinary tract, skin, or wound. Sometimes the temperature rises with the advent of raised intracranial pressure. The elevation varies with the suddenness and the severity of the rise in pressure, but is seldom an early change.

Nursing measures to reduce the raised temperature must be started as soon as an elevation is observed and continued until the temperature lowers and remains within normal limits. Cooling of the room, alcohol sponging, or the use of hypothermia blankets is frequently ordered if the patient is hyperthermic. Any special nursing measures or medications given should be charted on the patient's record.

Respiration

Maintenance of a clear airway is imperative in the management of neurosurgical patients. A lowering of the level of consciousness may be caused by a blocked airway because it aggravates raised intracranial pressure. To check whether an airway is clear, elevate the patient's chin and make sure the tongue is not blocking the airway. Listen for the *quiet* passage of air and watch for the *natural* movements of the chest. Do not be deceived by chest movements into assuming that the patient is actually ventilating; you may be observing respiratory movements which represent a struggle against a blocked airway. Observe and record the rate, rhythm, and type of respiration (e.g., shallow, stertorous, labored, or periodic). Watch for any evidence of respiratory distress, dyspnea, or cyanosis.

The patient should be placed in a semi-prone or lateral position with the head turned to the side and resting on a small pillow so that the mouth is at the outer edge of the pillow and pointing downward. This allows drainage of secretions and prevents the tongue from obstructing the airway. When the level of consciousness is depressed it may be necessary to remove secretions from the nose and mouth using a straight catheter and suction.

Seizures

The natural reaction to this symptom is an attempt to restrain the patient, but one cannot prevent the seizure from running its full course. The nurse should remain with the patient and send someone for assistance. The patient should be placed in lateral position, the head turned to the side and the chin pointing downward. This position allows maximum drainage of oral secretions and prevents the tongue from falling back and obstructing the airway. A mouth gag or any other device to hold the jaws apart is not recommended because while being inserted it may damage the teeth, gums, or tongue, yet do nothing to improve the airway. Remove the bedclothes from the patient in order to see exactly what parts of the body are involved in the seizure.

It is valuable if the nurse can witness the attack from its commencement, noting especially the way it begins and *the areas first involved.* To obtain an accurate description it may be necessary to jot down observations on scrap paper and later transfer them to the patient's record. Accuracy is important since the diagnosis of the condition often depends mainly on the nurse's description of the attack. Observations should include the following: onset of the seizure, the progress and sites involved, to which side the head and eyes turn, the level of consciousness, incontinence, duration, the condition of the patient after the seizure, and his ability to recall details.

SUMMARY

Recognition, interpretation, reporting and recording of the signs associated with increased intracranial pressure is the responsibility of the nurse. The management of the patient will vary with the cause. No matter what treatment is carried out, the cranio-cerebral testing must be continued until a normal level is established and maintained. In nursing neurosurgical patients the nurse must be familiar with the doctor's findings and his provisional diagnosis. She must determine the patient's base-line condition. By continuous monitoring of the symptoms and signs, the patient's condition is constantly compared with the base line already established; any deviations are reported at once. Effective action may depend on the accuracy and promptness with which the nurse recognizes abnormal developments and informs the doctor.

List the three most reliable signs related to neurological surgery.

What is the most important nursing accomplishment in caring for a neurological patient? Where have you heard this before?

List the equipment needed to effectively observe for neurological change.

List five levels of consciousness and give at least one means of evaluating this.

What should you look for and record when observing a seizure? How do you think you will react when observing your first seizure?

Describe how you would assess a patient's base line condition.

35.

Children's Reactions to Head Injuries

Kathryn R. Reeves

The following article illustrates the need for a good knowledge of growth and development. Lucky is the young patient who has a nurse who recognizes him to be a child and not a little adult. Read on to see how you can best individualize care for each of your young patients.

The section dealing with the typical changes that occur with increased intracranial pressure was omitted since the previous article by Jessie Young covers that subject. You may wish to read it first if you haven't already.

Pediatrics is not mini-medicine. It is not a scaled-down copy made of adult material. It is cut from totally different fabric. Since the child differs from the adult both anatomically and physiologically, different responses to disease, injury, and therapy can be expected. Evaluating such responses often must be done without help from the patient for the young child cannot describe changes occurring within his body.

Although norms have been established for various age groups, the individual child's behavior can be widely divergent, and still be normal. A two-year-old may be so well potty-trained that he will not use the bedpan; another may still be in diapers. Yet the nurse must have a good understanding of the normal child to be able to recognize clues that identify significant deviations.

In pediatric nursing, some variations of childhood behavior may not be significant. However, in some areas, observation of behavior traits can be critical.

This is particularly true in the care of the child with a head injury or other central nervous system disorder.

Evaluation of the behavior and physical reactions of neurologic patients plays a large role in pediatric nursing.

To limit guesswork in evaluating the neurologic state of young patients at the Childrens Hospital of Orange County, California, we have developed a questionnaire which is filled out by the parents of any child whose level of consciousness is of critical importance. There are four variations of the basic questionnaire, each with questions specific to four age groups. The information given in these questionnaires gives us a word picture of a child's normal activity level, both day and night. This is extremely helpful in evaluating his behavior and reactions in the hospital.

The manifestations of head injury in infants and children depend on the ways the injury occurred and what anatomic structures were damaged. Contrary to the adult's reactions to a relatively minor injury, a child tends to respond with severe and alarming signs and symptoms of unresponsiveness, vomiting, and shock.

CONCUSSION AND CONTUSION

Brain injuries, may or may not be associated with fractures of the skull. With the brief loss of consciousness in concussion there is no gross or microscopic evidence of injury to tissue. The patient regains consciousness, is in full control of himself, and knows what has happened to him. He may be "pseudo-shocky" immediately afterward, but this does not continue.

A contusion is a bruise of the brain, severe enough to rupture capillaries in the local area, and frequently is associated with laceration of the brain itself. The brain reacts to the injury and the scar it produces in much the same way as it reacts to a foreign body. The patient may lose consciousness and, if he wakes up, will show one or more signs of neurologic deficit, especially confusion which may subsequently clear over a period of time. He will usually have amnesia for events immediately preceding his accident as well as for the accident itself.

The protective response of the brain to injury often does the patient more harm than the injury. If blood is not getting to the tissue, for example, the body responds by sending more blood to the brain. With this compensating hyperemia, serum may ooze out into tissue, causing edema.

Although cerebral edema may occur in the first few hours after injury, it usually does not develop clinical significance early. For this reason, doctors hospitalize patients overnight for observation. Cerebral edema usually peaks in about 24 hours and the brain remains irritable for 72 hours.

COMMON SYMPTOMS

Common symptoms of head injury in children are headache, vertigo, and vomiting. A child who is too young to describe headache may show a characteristic type of restless irritability. A baby will be fussy and will resist being handled, but between episodes of headache he will be happy, alert, and normal. The presence of vertigo, which frequently occurs when the petrous bone has been fractured, can be suspected when the child assumes a position and vigorously resists efforts to move him from it. If forcibly moved, he often will vomit and show spontaneous nystagmus. Giddiness or unsteadiness, common in adults, is rare in children. Vomiting tends to occur more in mild, rather than in severe, injury.

Seizures as a result of head injury occur more frequently in children than in adults. Infants particularly may have short tonic seizures soon after a fall or a blow to the head, but subsequent recovery is often prompt. Although seizures caused by head injury may be of any variety, they are most often generalized regardless of the type of injury. Seizures which occur in the acute period of head injury rarely proceed into *status epilepticus* and do not seem to indicate an increased likelihood of chronic post-traumatic seizures.

Levels of consciousness are the single most important points of reference. However, nurses need to know what is "normal" for each child in order to give this basic information meaning. Our parent questionnaires in combination with the results of the initial examination are extremely valuable in helping us establish what is normal for each child.

Three of our former patients serve well to illustrate the value of the parent questionnaire.

Six-year-old Mark, admitted shortly after a "bicycle versus car" accident, quickly became alert and responsive, with no apparent ill effects. However, about 36 hours after admission, he woke screaming at 1:00 A.M. and seemed confused. He flailed out at the nurse, and then fell into a deep sleep. Although these signs may have indicated cerebral injury, his vital signs continued stable, and a check of the questionnaire showed his mother's comment, "Always has nightmares and cries out at night and thrashes around." Mark, we decided, was reacting normally.

Kelly, a five-year-old girl, also seemed normal after admission following a fall in the bathtub. Although she had had several episodes of vomiting, her vital signs were stable. One hour after bedtime (and about eight hours postaccident) the aide reported that, although Kelly could be aroused by shaking, she had been incontinent. The nurse noted that the mother had written on the questionnaire "Kelly never (not even rarely) wets the bed." This alerted us to the possibility of cerebral dysfunction. On examination the doctor found early signs of increasing cerebral edema and prescribed intravenous Mannitol 20 percent immediately. In addition, Decadron was given intramuscularly to reduce inflammation and edema, and phenobarbital (also given intramuscularly) to reduce the possibility of seizures. Twelve hours later, because there was still evidence of cerebral edema she received another course of Mannitol. The Decadron was gradually decreased, then discontinued, and by the time of her discharge she was being maintained on a prophylactic dose of oral phenobarbital. In this case, the early discovery of cerebral edema resulted in successful treatment with medication, reducing the possibility of further brain trauma.

Another victim of an automobile accident was three-year-old Michael. He had sustained some cerebral contusion, had a lowered level of consciousness, and was disoriented for several days. His condition slowly improved, and when he began to talk he used the hesitant, "scanning" speech that is indicative of cerebellar involvement. However, his mother's description of his speech on the questionnaire was "slow and slurred," and later, when she was visiting, she said he was talking as he always did. Although his speech was "normal" for him, it was still abnormal, so after his recovery we referred him to the outpatient speech clinic.

An added bonus to our use of the questionnaire has been an increased awareness on the part of the nursing staff regarding the responsibility of accurate and knowledgeable observation and charting*

*Copies of the questionnaires described in this article are available from the author.

How does the child's reaction to minor head injury compare with that of an adult?

How could you get information from patients if there were no questionnaires available? What questions would need to be included? How would these questions probably change for the following age groups: 1 to 3, 5 to 9, 11 to 14, and 15 to 20?

36.

The Drops of Life: Fluids and Electrolytes

Margaret A. Berry
Colette B. Kerlin

Thirst, perspiration, and dry, chapped lips are well-known signs of the body's reaction to fluids. How does this happen? What is the significance to the nurse and the patient? These two articles and especially the chart on pages 242-243 should be referred to as you care for patients with fluid and electrolyte disturbances.

Nurses play a crucial role in preventing fluid and electrolyte imbalance. They are with the patient 24 hours a day. By charting intake and output, and observing the patient closely for signs and symptoms, they can prevent imbalance in many cases. If it occurs, they can help prevent further imbalance and thus contribute to the prevention of further pathology. Surely there is no more essential nursing task, or one of greater service to the patient!

HOMEOSTASIS: KEY TO IMBALANCE

Though man lives a terrestial existence, at the cellular level he is still aquatic. Water accounts for 60 to 70 per cent of the body weight. Aqueous solutions constantly bathe the body cells as well as carry waste substances from them to the removal organs (kidneys, G.I. tract, skin, lungs). Suspended in these solutions are *electrolytes.*

Electrolytes are particles resulting from the breakdown of inorganic compounds. The most important ones in the body are sodium, potassium, calcium, magnesium, chloride, phosphate, and bicarbonate. These dissolve in the body fluids as *ions* that carry either a positive electrical charge (cation) or a negative charge (anion).

Water and electrolytes maintain a homeostatic relationship. *Homeostasis* implies a state of dynamic equilibrium in which the components of body fluids are constantly changing yet remain the same in volume, pH (hydrogen ion concentration), and chemical composition. To maintain homeostasis, positive and negative ions reach a balance at which they cancel out each other's attraction.

There are two kinds of body fluids: *intracellular* and *extracellular* (includes the blood). Both contain similar electrolytes but in different concentrations. For example, the intracellular fluid is high in potassium, low in sodium; the extracellular fluid is high in sodium, low in potassium.

Water and electrolytes readily pass through the cell's semipermeable membrane, thus providing nourishment and removing wastes. In illness, the process may become unbalanced. For instance, excessive sodium ions may concentrate in the extracellular fluid of a tissue. Water then migrates there in large amounts to dilute the sodium and equalize the pH between intracellular and extracellular fluid. Edema results.

MAINTAINING FLUID BALANCE

This is the nurse's first and, perhaps, greatest concern. These are some facts to keep in mind:

Normally, an adult exchanges about 2,750 ml. of fluid in each 24-hour period. This is usually ingested as 1,650 ml. of frank fluids (water, coffee, juice, etc.) and 750 ml. in foods (preformed water). In addition, about 350 ml. is derived from oxidative metabolism. The total is excreted as follows: about 1,700 ml. in the urine, 500 ml. through normal respiration, 400 ml. through normal perspiration, and 150 ml. in the feces.

To help maintain adequate intake and output, the nurse routinely elicits from each patient a history of his drinking and eating patterns. She is not content simply to offer the usual pitcher of water and refresh it on schedule or demand. When forced fluids are indicated, she offers favorite foods as well as drinks between meals. Salads, gelatin desserts, fruits, and soups all help to reduce the need to force fluids. (Green and leafy vegetables are 96 to 98 per cent water.)

Secondly, she observes the patient closely for unusual fluid loss. Obvious loss may occur through vomiting, diarrhea, hemorrhage, and drainage; less obviously, through mouth breathing, perspiring, excessive talking, and increased respiration.

She also observes for early signs of imbalance. For example, unusual thirst, dry skin and mucous membranes, and constipation may be subtle indications of impending dehydration. Other signs, less subtle, include increased pulse and

Water and Electrolyte Imbalances

Substance	Major Functions	Effects of Too Little	Effects of Too Much	Primary Food Sources
Water	Medium of body fluids, chemical changes, body temperature; lubricant	Observable symptoms: highly concentrated urine, oliguria, thirst, fever. Others: increase in serum solute and sodium concentration, circulatory failure	Observable symptoms: dilute urine, polyuria, headache, confusion, nausea, vomiting, weakness, muscle twitching and cramps, convulsions, coma. Others: decrease in serum solute and sodium concentration, increase in intracranial pressure	All liquids, fruits, vegetables, eggs, meat
Sodium	Osmotic pressure, muscle and nerve irritability	Observable symptoms: hypotension, nausea, vomiting, diarrhea, headache, muscle weakness, abdominal cramps. Others: decrease in extracellular fluid volume, hemoconcentration, loss of tissue elasticity, microcardia	Observable symptoms: manic excitement, tachycardia, edema. Others: increase in extracellular fluid, congestive heart failure, tendency to potassium deficiency	Salt, meat, fish, fowl, milk, cheese, eggnog, tomato juice, bread, butter, cereals, pickles, cola beverages
Potassium	Intracellular fluid balance, regular heart rhythm, muscle and nerve irritability	Observable symptoms: apathy or apprehension lethargy, muscle weakness, nausea, tachycardia. Others: ileus or diarrhea, hypopotassemia, metabolic alkalosis	Observable symptoms: muscle weakness, nausea, colic, diarrhea, changes in ECG. Others: hyperpotassium, cardiac arrest	Meat, fish, fowl, cereals, fruit, juices (grape, apple, cranberry, orange, pear, apricot), bananas, tea, cola beverages

Water and Electrolyte Imbalances *(Continued)*

Substance	Major Functions	Effects of Too Little	Effects of Too Much	Primary Food Sources
Calcium	Muscle contraction, normal heart rhythm, nerve irritability, blood clotting	Observable symptoms: numbness tingling of nose, ears, finger tips, or toes; tetany	Few clinical problems	Milk, cottage cheese, ice cream, broccoli, shrimp
Magnesium	Muscle and nerve irritability	Observable symptoms: hypotonic tetany. Others: fibrillary muscle twitching	Few clinical problems	Milk, cereals
Chloride	Osmotic pressure	Occur only after prolonged vomiting; few clinical problems	Few clinical problems	Salt, milk, eggnog
Phosphate	Building of bones and teeth, buffering system, transport of fatty acids, metabolizing of fats and carbohydrates	Hypophosphatemia, poor mineralization of bones, rickets	Observable symptom: tetany. Others: hyperphosphatemia, hypocalcemia	Milk, egg yolk, whole-grain cereals
Bicarbonate	Acid-base balance	Ketosis augmentation of protoplasmic catabolism, tendency to greater water and electrolyte losses	Hyperglycemia, hepatic failure	Eggs, meat, beef broth, fish, poultry chicken broth

respiration, decreased urinary output, highly concentrated urine, fever, and weight loss.

When observing for signs of fluid retention, the nurse keeps in mind that retention is usually caused by problems of excretion rather than by malfunctioning of the fluid-electrolyte mechanism. She regularly examines the most dependent parts of the body for signs of edema. (For the patient on bed rest, the buttocks are more susceptible than feet and ankles.) She may weigh the patient each morning before fluid and food intake, and watch for a small but steady weight gain. She is alert for signs of headache and mental confusion, as these may signal fluid retention in the central nervous system and could lead to idiopathic coma and/or convulsions.

MAINTAINING ELECTROLYTE BALANCE

Because of homeostasis, fluid balance and electrolyte balance are interdependent. For instance, when fluids become trapped in tissues or organs — as in cases of wound-swelling, edema, ascites, or intestinal obstruction — electrolytes trapped in the fluids are not available for normal distribution, and the patient may suffer from electrolyte imbalance as well as fluid imbalance. Similarly, when there is excessive electrolyte loss, there is excessive fluid loss.

But electrolyte imbalance is much more complex than a simple relationship with the gross amount of fluids. For example, if the kidneys become diseased so that they cannot excrete normal amounts of sodium, they will not excrete normal amounts of water either. Sodium has an indirect relationship with potassium, also. When sodium levels in the extracellular fluids go up, potassium levels go down. Even prolonged stress can cause electrolyte imbalance as a response to adrenal-cortical activity.

To help maintain electrolyte balance, the nurse needs a working knowledge of the electrolytes and their characteristics, intake sources and output routes, and kinds of illnesses and situations that make a patient vulnerable to imbalance. As with fluid balance, she observes the patient closely for excessive loss and signs of imbalance.

Electrolytes normally enter the body as foods. They leave with the body fluids, sometimes in varying proportions. For instance, quantities of all electrolytes are lost in excessive salivation, vomiting, or diarrhea. With excessive perspiration, sodium is the major loss.

A balanced diet is usually adequate to maintain electrolyte balance. However, if an imbalance of a specific electrolyte is known or suspected, foods rich in that substance may be given. For example, the nurse who notes from lab reports that a patient's potassium level is low may give him extra portions of grape juice, say, or add bananas to his diet. If the potassium level continues to drop, the physician may have to order potassium iodide or chloride, given orally or I.V.

Certain symptoms are peculiar to each electrolyte imbalance, whether a deficit or an excess. The symptoms and related information for the seven common electrolytes are provided in the accompanying table. By observing and reporting early symptoms, the nurse can alert the doctor to the possible need for diagnosis and treatment, including blood studies and the administration of additives or replacements.

If it becomes necessary to give an electrolyte solution intravenously, the nurse bears in mind that it must be given at a moderate rate so that the body's normal regulating mechanism can achieve a physiological balance. Thus she monitors the flow carefully.

To Summarize

Maintaining hydration and electrolyte balance is an important aspect of skilled nursing care. Through her knowledge of entry and exit patterns and of the situations that make a patient prone to fluid and electrolyte problems, the nurse can help prevent further pathology. When she makes effective use of careful observation combined with knowledge, it may be unnecessary for the doctor to order "Force fluids" or "I.V.s," and the patient is the winner.

37.

Fluids and Electrolytes

Richard E. Burgess

Rachel Carson, talking about evolutionary processes in *The Sea Around Us,* wrote: "When they went ashore the animals that took up a land life carried with them a part of the sea in their bodies, a heritage which they passed on to their children and which even today links each land animal with its origin in the ancient sea.*

CLINICAL SIGNIFICANCE

Let's look at the difference in the total body water of infants in comparison to adults — 75 percent in contrast to 60 percent. It is thought that this extra water in infants acts as a protective mechanism, compensating for their larger surface area in relation to body weight. The actual amount of fluid and electrolyte in an infant is quite small.

Obviously, in parenteral therapy of infants and young children, much smaller quantities must be carefully given at a slower rate. This is necessary to prevent overexpanding the vascular space or overtaxing the homeostatic mechanisms which normally regulate the distribution and composition of the body fluids.

Of great clinical significance is the maintenance of proper volume and electrolyte composition within the fluid spaces. Serious fluid and electrolyte imbalance may result whenever there is either too much or too little of one or more electrolytes, or of water, in a space. This may also happen when there is a shift of water or electrolytes from one space to another.

Let's look at potassium, for instance, which has been receiving considerable

*CARSON, RACHEL. *The Sea Around Us.* New York, New American Library, 1961, p. 28.

attention during the past few years. Potassium plays an important role in many intracellular processes; over 98 percent of the body's total potassium is *within* the cells. When tissues are destroyed as a result of trauma, starvation, or wasting diseases, large amounts of potassium are released. This excess potassium is excreted in the urine if kidney function is normal; if it is not, the potassium piles up in the extracellular fluid, with potentially serious results.

On the other hand, when potassium is lost from the body because of vomiting, diarrhea, or use of diuretics, the kidney conserves potassium. Despite this action on the kidney's part, however, the patient with potassium loss may require extra amounts of potassium by infusion, especially if he cannot tolerate an adequate oral intake. The parenteral potassium is necessary to replace excessive losses of this substance, to meet daily needs for it, and to build new tissue.

The importance of adequate kidney function during potassium administration cannot be overemphasized. Otherwise, excessive quantities of potassium can accumulate in the plasma and cause cardiac arrhythmias and death. Kidney function is usually evaluated before potassium administration by rapidly infusing 500 to 1,000 ml. of a solution such as 5 percent dextrose in 0.2 percent sodium chloride. If diuresis occurs in less than an hour, then a multiple electrolyte solution containing adequate maintenance or replacement quantities of potassium as well as of other electrolytes may be safely administered.

Sodium, as we have seen, is contained mostly within the extracellular compartment. One of its main functions is to influence the distribution and quantity of water in the body. This maintenance of a proper concentration and volume of the extracellular fluid is very important. The blood volume and heart output, and hence the total circulation, are dependent on this vital reservoir. In the course of geologic history, physiologic mechanisms have evolved which enable the kidney to either conserve or excrete sodium and water. This happens normally whenever there are changes in extracellular fluid volume, blood volume, or cardiac output. Thus, when sodium is lost from the body after vomiting, diarrhea, or severe sweating, there is a reduction in extracellular fluid and plasma volume. This may lead to impaired renal and circulatory function until the losses are replaced. However, in salt-retaining patients with heart, liver, or kidney disease, this replacement must be done judiciously to avoid the production of edema.

Most laboratory analyses of electrolyte content are carried out on the plasma, which represents less than one twelfth of the total body fluid. The results may occasionally be misleading since, like the top of an iceberg extending above the sea, the plasma may give only a hint of what lies beneath.

Electrolyte determinations of plasma sometimes may actually misrepresent conditions in the other spaces. For example, the plasma of a very edematous cardiac patient may show a reduced serum sodium concentration despite the existence of an enormous excess of total body sodium. This is because in severe heart failure in patients on low sodium diets, water may be retained in excess of sodium. This dilutes the concentration of all electrolytes in body fluids.

PARENTERAL THERAPY

For correct therapeutic management, therefore, chemical analyses of the plasma and urine must be correlated with the clinical history and findings.

To meet water, electrolyte, and a small part of the caloric needs, a multiple electrolyte *maintenance* solution with dextrose or other carbohydrate is usually given after determination of adequate urine formation. Dosage is calculated on the basis of the body's need for water. Kidney function is depended upon to eliminate any small excesses of electrolyte.

The third reason for parenteral fluid and electrolyte therapy is to replace losses which may be occurring at the moment as a result of diarrhea, vomiting, a draining fistula, gastric suction, and the like. A *replacement* solution with an electrolyte content similar to that of the fluid being lost is usually given, in amounts approximately equal to the volume lost.

Many of these solutions are commercially available, developed from formulas calculated to meet specific types of needs. Thus, there are maintenance solutions for both adults and children, gastric replacement solutions for use in instances of long continued gastric suction, and a solution whose formula closely resembles the electrolyte content of blood plasma and which is used to expand the volume of the vascular space. This last solution, with perhaps additional potassium, may also be used to replace losses from diarrhea.

Solutions may also be "tailor made" within the hospital to meet individual needs. Thus, 5 or 10 percent carbohydrate in water, with appropriate added electrolytes (these are available, in concentrated form, in vials), might be used to make up a maintenance or replacement solution.

The nurse has many responsibilities in parenteral therapy, especially when there are serious fluid and electrolyte imbalances. Often, she is the one who starts the infusion; nearly always, she is the one who monitors its progress. She must keep careful records of what the patient is receiving and assume responsibility for accurate intake-output figures. Equally important, she must be alert to signs of imbalance — developing edema, for instance, or the nausea, muscular weakness, and mental depression which may indicate potassium deficiency. The presence of symptoms like these may very well indicate the need for an adjustment in therapy.

CONDITIONS OF IMBALANCE

These illustrative examples of imbalance are somewhat oversimplified, since actual cases are often a combination of several conditions interacting with each other. Nevertheless, they do clarify the basic principles that have been discussed.

Dehydration

Simple dehydration can result from fever, sweating, or insufficient water intake. Water and a little electrolyte are needed to correct it.

Water Intoxication

This condition of excessive total body water is the reverse of the previous example. It may result, among other causes, from repeated tap water enemas or from excess water given either orally or intravenously (5 percent dextrose without sodium chloride, for instance) to patients losing electrolyte during gastric suction, vomiting, or diarrhea. With the increased amount of water, the electrolyte concentration in the body fluids is reduced.

The aim in treatment is to promote water excretion and reduce water intake. If the concentrations of electrolytes in the plasma are very low, solutions containing relatively high concentrations of sodium chloride are given. In less severe cases water restriction may be sufficiently effective, or an extracellular replacement solution may be given. These actions raise extracellular electrolyte concentrations, drawing water out of the cells and increasing urine output.

Sodium Excess

This may develop in the patient who has cardiac, renal, or liver disease which interferes with his elimination of salt, especially if he has been given excessive quantities of sodium solutions. The result is expanded extracellular fluid volume, or edema, as the excess salt holds the fluid there. The fluid volume within the cells does not change, however.

Treatment of this imbalance aims at reducing the intake of salt and water while the kidneys eliminate the overload of electrolytes and water from the plasma. Diuretics are given to increase sodium excretion. Potassium solutions, or special combinations of electrolytes, may be ordered later to correct cellular deficiencies which developed during imbalance.

Burns

After a burn, there is a large shift of fluid and electrolytes from the plasma to the interstitial spaces of the burned areas. With the resultant lowered blood volume, shock impends, the kidneys begin to shut down, and potassium may accumulate to dangerous levels in the plasma.

The shock must first be combated by introducing large volumes of colloids such as dextran or plasma into the vascular compartment. Since these substances pass only with great difficulty through the capillary wall, they help to hold fluid within this compartment. If the burn is severe, whole blood may be needed. Lactated Ringer's solution with 5 percent dextrose is also used to provide water and some electrolytes, and to minimize the development of acidosis.

Later, during the healing phase, the fluid shifts back into the plasma. At this time, oral or intravenous fluids should be reduced while the kidneys catch up and eliminate any excess quantities of water and electrolytes.

These, then, are some examples of fluid and electrolyte imbalances and their causes, and of the ways in which informed nursing observation, as well as monitoring of therapy, can enable the body's homeostatic mechanisms to regain and carry out their function.

List some signs and symptoms of fluid and electrolyte imbalance. Which would involve intracellular fluid excess? Which would include extra-cellular excess?

Why would sodium bicarbonate be added to an I.V. solution being given to a patient with diabetes?

Add, in writing, the ways each substance listed on the chart (pages 242-243) enters and leaves the body and what health problems make a person prone to fluid and electrolyte imbalance.

PREVENTING

38.
Perineal Care of the Incapacitated Patient

Gertrude E. Gibbs

If you have read about touching in "Maternal Touch" you may be able to recognize your own behavior as you visualize yourself giving perineal care to a patient. Are you a fingertip nurse? Think about your patient's feelings about touch – the helpless patient who has come to terms with touch needs you. If you do not know what perineal care is, read the following article.

Perineal care is an aspect of daily patient care that has often been neglected, not only in practice but even in theory.

It is easy to understand how this came about. In our culture, sex is a subject that has always generated anxiety and even now is not often discussed freely and without embarrassment. The perineal area, because of its anatomic link with sexual activity, was therefore also not discussed.

The first sign of poor perineal care is a fetid odor noticeable when the patient's bedcovers are lifted. My experience has been that many patients feel very uncomfortable about the odor and say so. Further signs of neglect might be discharge and skin breakdown. As always, nursing prevention is much simpler than cure. Poor perineal care has also been blamed for the high incidence of bladder infection in patients with indwelling catheters. Patients with indwelling catheters need the same, or more frequent, perineal care than patients without them.

FOR FEMALE PATIENTS

The procedure I use for giving perineal care to female patients is very similar to the cleansing done prior to catheterization. I place a bath towel lengthwise under the patient's hips so that one end can be used for drying the perineum and the other end, later, for drying the anal region. Then I drape the patient with a bath blanket, covering her flexed legs. I use cotton balls and hexachlorophene with warm water, and clear warm water for rinsing. I use one cotton ball each time to wipe from the pubis to the perirectal area, then discard the cotton into a plastic bag. (Since cotton balls stop up the plumbing, they should be discarded with paper trash.)

First, the outer perineum and area between thighs and labia are washed well, then dried and powered. I use a cotton ball as a powder puff to avoid caking of powder in the skin creases. With obese patients it is very difficult to cleanse this area adequately but, since these patients are prone to perspire profusely, washing must not be neglected. Then the labia are separated, and the labia minora are washed inside on each side, over the urinary meatus and vaginal orifice, again using a separate cotton ball for each downward stroke and wiping purposefully from front to back. This area is rinsed in the same manner with warm water and dried with the towel.

Then I place the patient on her side, separate the buttocks, and wash the posterior area, with special attention to the anal region. Here again I use disposable material for washing — cotton balls, tissue, or even clean rags if the area is very soiled. It seems to me very poor technique to use a washcloth, soil it with stool, then rinse it in the washbasin and use it and the water again. After drying the skin I might apply powder, white petrolatum, or zinc oxide, depending on the condition of the skin. When patients are washed in this way with their bath, odors are eliminated and comfort is enhanced. This is one area that should not be neglected, and the patient should receive this care even if time is short.

FOR MALE PATIENTS

When giving perineal care to a male patient I drape him and arrange the bath towel lengthwise as described earlier. The penis should be washed first. In the uncircumcised male the foreskin should be pulled back and then the glans and the reflecting surface of the prepuce washed and dried. If the foreskin is not pulled back, smegma accumulates. This is a good medium for bacterial growth and also causes an offensive odor. The foreskin then should be pulled back over the end of the penis to prevent constriction, which could lead to edema and subsequent inability to void. (If paraphimosis occurs, it can be a surgical emergency.)

Next, the outside of the foreskin and penis is washed, including the posterior side. To wash the scrotum, the patient's legs should be well separated and the scrotum lifted up and forward. The anterior and posterior sides are washed, and the thighs are cleansed at this time, also. As with any skin surfaces, these reflecting and opposing skin areas, if not properly cared for, can easily become excoriated. All areas need to be rinsed well, dried, and powder applied sparingly with a cotton ball. Then the patient is turned to his side, his buttocks are separated, and the area from scrotum to anus washed, dried, and powdered.

When washing the genitalia, long swift strokes should be employed. This area is very sensitive and the patient may have an erection. When this happened to a patient being bathed by one of my students, a motherly practical nurse who had three grown boys of her own, she simply left the room and returned later to complete the bath. Yet in writing about her experience, this student — middle-aged, married, and a mother of sons — mentioned her embarrassment. How would a young nursing student feel in such a situation if this possibility is not discussed beforehand?

Another solution is to ignore the erection and complete the bath. However, if either the patient or the nurse is too embarrassed, it would be better for her to leave. Yet another suggestion is to wash the scrotum first and leave the washing of the penis until last, since it is manipulation of the penis that is most likely to cause an erection. In this case, if the scrotum is not clean the water should be changed, and perhaps a fresh washcloth used.

When I give perineal care I wear disposable gloves. Apparently this is controversial. The faction against gloves claims that their use makes the patient feel as if he were dirty and that we do not like to touch him. I claim this is true. In this area the patient *is* "dirty" from a bacteriologic point of view. Otherwise, why would we spend so much time and effort educating children and food handlers to wash their hands well after using the toilet? To me, it is important that patients receive the much needed perineal care, and whether the patient feels the nurse is showing distaste depends on the nurse's real attitude, not on whether or not she wears gloves. If she is natural and approaches this whole procedure matter-of-factly without distaste, her conscientiousness about his care is communicated, not the details of her technique.

Did you encounter any new words? How about labia, fetid, catheriza-
tion, urinary, meatus, perineum, glans, prepuce, foreskin, smegma, and
paraphimosis? Look them up if you are unsure of their meaning.

Discuss the method of giving perineal care, described here, with your
instructor. How do you feel about cleansing a patient with or without
gloves on your hands? What concerns do you have when giving male
pericare?

Review this article as a soon-to-be-graduate of a nursing program and
evaluate the change in your feelings.

Describe five different patients who should have "pericare" added to
their nursing care plans.

SUPPORTING

39.
What to Do About Thirst

Mary Fenton

From reading the preceding articles, you know that fluids and electrolytes are not only necessary to life but must be in balance. What can be done for the thirsty patient who is NPO or on restricted fluids? In the following article, read to find out about thirst, what it is, and why it occurs; then list some of the theories. Relate what you read to your own feelings of thirst and what you do to quench your thirst as you begin to understand its physiology.

Everyone gets thirsty from time to time and relieves the sensation by taking something to drink. In other words, thirst is a normal symptom in the healthy person, whose fluid intake is generally regulated by (1) the intensity of his thirst, and (2) his normal pattern of fluid intake. This pattern, in time, may be determined by his inherent physiologic makeup — which may vary from one person to another — or, even more probable, by environmental or cultural factors.

In the hospital patient, however, thirst is often created by the restriction of fluids associated with the treatment of such conditions as renal or cardiac failure. In these situations thirst cannot be relieved by the normal and obvious means of increasing the fluid intake. The nurse's responsibility, therefore, is to maintain the restricted fluids regimen and at the same time promote the patient's comfort and well-being. Thirst *can* be dealt with effectively if the nurse understands why thirst occurs and is familiar with the nursing principles on which her intervention to relieve it can be based.

PHYSIOLOGY OF THIRST

There are many theories to explain the mechanism of thirst and factors related to it. As early as 1918 Cannon proposed that the thirst of dehydration could be explained on the basis of decreased salivary flow and associated drying of the mouth.

There is a difference, however, between the decrease in salivary flow and resulting dry mouth engendered by dehydration, and the dryness of the mouth that may result from such other oral factors as disagreeable taste, ingestion of salty food or candy, drying of the mouth by nasal oxygen or mouth breathing, and certain drugs such as atropine. These factors, too, may lead to increased fluid intake, even though a patient's hydration is adequate.

Holmes has observed reductions in salivary flow and presumed dryness of the mouth in clinical situations such as renal or cardiac failure where thirst or increased fluid intake were important considerations in the patient's management. Upon questioning, these patients revealed that much of their drinking was related to their desire to relieve the discomfort of a dry mouth, peculiar taste, or a "cottony" feeling. There is also evidence that thirst or a desire for water can be experienced even when the mouth is wet; under these circumstances, mere wetting of the mouth does not give relief. It is possible, then, that the salivary glands do not always play a major role in the thirst mechanism.

Gilman has suggested that intracellular dehydration is the primary tissue factor in the stimulation of the thirst mechanism, and he therefore postulates that drinking behavior is directed toward the replenishment of body water. Other studies have shown that an increase in osmotic pressure of the blood (hyperosmolality associated with hypernatremia) will likewise decrease the salivary flow and lead to a dry mouth, resulting in the sensation of thirst. Finally, the recognized thirst of hemorrhage and shock is associated with significant reductions in plasma and blood volume; the continued presence of thirst in such situations is assumed to be a definite indication of undertreatment of the condition.

Probably both oral and gastric factors play a major role in the satisfaction of thirst. Holding water in the mouth will relieve thirst for about 15 minutes; however, such "sham drinking" of water that does not enter the stomach provides only temporary relief. Gastric distention *per se* will relieve thirst for about one to two hours. This distention lengthens the intervals between drinking periods, but permanent satiety depends ultimately upon the absorption of water from the gastrointestinal tract.

Many patients maintained in perfect fluid balance by intravenous therapy will still complain of severe thirst. Furthermore, many inappropriate increases in fluid intake occur in patients who have had gastric resection or pathology of the stomach. All these factors have practical significance when one is attempting to relieve thirst in the presence of a restricted fluid intake.

Probably the most common "thirsty" patient is the one with renal or cardiac failure who is experiencing thirst because of a restricted fluid intake and accompanying oral factors. Nursing intervention must, of course, be individualized for each patient, but six main factors should be taken into consideration in planning care: *fluid intake, condition of the oral cavity, output* or *fluid loss, diet, motor ability,* and the patient's *mental state.* With information about these factors, care can then be planned around the patient's individual pattern of fluid intake, his medical regimen, including the diet and amount and type of fluid allowed, and his physical and mental state.

In most situations the nurse must work within the limits of the amount and type of fluid prescribed for, or allowed, the patient. Essential to her nursing care plan, therefore, must be knowledge of the patient's normal and hospital drinking patterns: when, how much, and what he drinks, the amount he takes with meals and medications, and so on.

FLUID INTAKE

Holmes has suggested that fluid intake, to a large degree, may relate to a long-established drinking pattern. Thus, if the nurse learns that a patient is accustomed to drinking large amounts of coffee in the morning or throughout the day, or if he usually consumes large amounts of fluid at mealtime, she may have to try to institute a new pattern of fluid intake in the hospital. Fluids with meals may need to be limited, so that the total liquid may be spread more evenly throughout other times of the day and night. This is especially important if the patient tends to wake up frequently and complain of thirst.

Some patients may be in the habit of taking a whole glass of water at a time, regardless of how much they actually want. In this situation, only small amounts of fluid should be offered; the use of a small glass helps, too. The optical illusion provided by large glasses with small capacities is another aid.

The taste of the water — and this may vary greatly from one locale to another — is another consideration. A patient unaccustomed to the taste of the hospital water may not find it satisfying. If the water contains substantial amounts of chlorine, letting it stand for eight hours may make it more palatable and therefore more satisfying.

Holmes also found that fluids consumed with medication could account for a significant portion of the total allowed fluid. This represents a therapeutic problem in patients on restricted fluids. Two major factors which determined the amount of fluid taken with medication were the frequency of administration and the way the medication tasted to the patient.

Although the physician determines the frequency of medications, it is often the nurse who determines the schedule for giving them. Therefore, the more medicines that can be given safely at the same time, the smaller the total fluid taken with medications.

The total number of pills or capsules has been found to be less important in relation to the amount of fluid ingested than the size of the pills or capsules. Many patients have difficulty swallowing large pills, especially when their mouths are dry, and naturally require more water to wash them down. Substituting several small pills for one large one whenever possible is another way to reduce the fluid taken with medications. Giving medications at mealtime also cuts down the amount of fluid.

A medication's taste may influence the amount of fluid that is taken with it, especially if the medication is in liquid form. If possible, capsules or pills should be substituted; otherwise, an attempt should be made to disguise the taste in an appropriate vehicle.

The temperature of the water is another factor. Some patients tend to take less when it is cold, and the nurse should keep this in mind.

ORAL CAVITY

The color, turgor, and intactness of the mucous membranes, gums, and tongue will help the nurse to assess the condition of the oral cavity. The presence of salivary flow and the ability to swallow are also relevant. A "dry" mouth, even though induced by factors other than restricted fluid intake, will also create a desire for fluid.

Sometimes the dryness is due to such factors as the administration of nasal oxygen, dyspnea, or mouth breathing. Under these circumstances, increased humidification of the air and oxygen and frequent cleansing and lubrication of the mouth with a half and half mixture of lemon juice and glycerine will provide some relief.

Dryness of the mouth may also be associated with a reduction in salivary flow such as occurs in patients with renal or cardiac failure. In either condition, relieving the thirst and providing appropriate mouth care are important nursing problems. To decrease the incidence of parotitis, gum chewing can be instituted to stimulate salivary flow. And all possible measures to keep the mouth moist and clean and thereby reduce thirst must be taken, since an increase in fluid intake could be serious.

OUTPUT OR FLUID LOSS

As every nurse knows, the balance between intake and output is important if the desired state of hydration is to be maintained and any necessary fluid replacement to be accurately determined. Otherwise, a patient might suffer from continuing and unnecessary thirst, simply because his fluid losses were not recognized.

This calls for accurate measurement not only of urinary output but also of fluid lost through vomiting, diarrhea, and diaphoresis (often due to a temperature elevation). Perspiration may also be induced by the temperature and humidity of the patient's room — factors that the nurse should control accordingly.

There may also be insensible fluid loss as a result of increased or difficult respirations. In practically all instances, daily weights are indicated to determine whether the patient is maintaining the prescribed fluid balance.

DIET

Often, when a patient is on restricted fluids, he will also be on some sort of therapeutic or restricted diet. Any type of dietary restriction usually results in a less palatable diet and one that may contain dry, thirst-producing foods; mashed potatoes are one common example.

Special diets should therefore be carefully checked for dry foods and, whenever possible, moist foods should be substituted. These, obviously, require less fluid to wash down. Salty foods, candy, and sugar solutions are likely to produce thirst, so their presence in the diet should also be checked.

The gastric distention that follows a meal, however, will inhibit thirst. Encouraging the patient to eat, therefore, will not only be an aid to nutrition but may also help to relieve thirst.

Fatty foods are less likely than others to produce oral discomfort. Mixing the patient's allotted fat with other foods is another way to decrease his desire for fluid with the meal.

MOTOR ABILITY

Can the patient reach out and pour himself a glass of water? Or walk down the hall to the drinking fountain? If he can, it may become more difficult to control and keep track of his fluid intake. Obviously, careful explanation of why his fluid intake must be regulated is indicated. In addition, utilization of the thirst-relieving measures already described may help a great deal in this situation.

MENTAL STATE

The patient's orientation to time, place, and person, his intellectual and educational level, and his ability to understand his disease and the reason his fluids are restricted may also influence the comfort and success of a limited fluid regimen and the patient's adherence to it. Depending on the above factors, one form or another of diversional therapy might be instituted to focus the patient's mind on something other than his thirst. The patient on limited fluids who is confined to bed day after day with nothing to do may just lie there and think about how thirsty he is — and keep begging the nursing staff for water which, unfortunately, he cannot have.

One such patient with renal failure was restricted to 500 cc. of fluid per 24 hours. Cared for on a large open ward, he kept constantly asking the nursing staff, the other patients, and even the visitors for water. Even though the reason for restricting his fluids had been explained to him again and again, he was becoming confused and agitated and could concentrate only on his thirst and desire for water. This situation went on for several days until a nursing aide happened to give him a magazine to read. He immediately became engrossed in it and did not request any water while he was reading, which lasted for the rest of the afternoon.

Observing this happy result, the nursing staff kept him supplied with something to read from then on. The arrival of a television set on the ward occupied even more of his time and attention, so that his craving for water became much less of a problem. He stayed on his restricted fluid therapy for the rest of his hospitalization, and his spirits improved considerably.

Give an example of how culture, environment, and physical makeup may affect a person's fluid intake. What other factors influence this?

List some specific examples how you could increase a thirsty patient's comfort even though he is on restricted fluids.

40.

Hospital Food Can Help or Hinder Care

Majorie E. Newton
Jeannette Folta

*Patients often spend more time talking about food than any other
subject and it seems that nurses spend the least time and effort
helping patients meet their nutritional needs in comparison to their
other needs. It is difficult to find written records of food
consumed or methods employed to improve nutritional intake. This
may be because nurses are not involved in preparing the food or
because nutritional status is difficult to evaluate and follow its
changes. Whatever the reasons, this article will give those nurses
who are interested several ways to make eating more enjoyable in a
hospital, and some clues as to why a patient may not be eating and
drinking.*

Food is important to all of us — not just the kind and amount of food we eat,
but when we eat as well.

We cannot assume that the patient who doesn't eat simply has no appetite or
doesn't like the food. We need to recognize that patients respond to food in light
of their own values and cultural patterns.

In most hospitals, we could make better use of social science concepts to
understand the significance of eating behaviors.

For example, the average American pattern of eating is a rather light to
medium breakfast on arising, a coffee break at midmorning, a light lunch
perhaps, a coffee break, a heavy dinner, and a bedtime snack of anything from
popcorn to pizza.

Contrast this with the pattern of a Frenchman, who is accustomed to cocoa and perhaps a sweet roll when he arises, followed at 10:00 A.M. by the equivalent of a fair-sized lunch or later by a heavy lunch. On the other hand, a person of Slavic origin may be used to two big meals a day.

In the average hospital, however, the custom is to serve a regular breakfast from one to three hours after patients are awakened, a rather heavy meal at noon, and a light supper. Patients may get crackers or cookies and milk at bedtime.

The size of portions served in hospitals may be another source of difficulty. A physical laborer used to eating 5,000 calories or more daily may feel resentful and deprived, and a petite, retired woman, who is used to small meals, may feel overwhelmed when confronted with the size of hospital portions and meals.

Eating is a social situation, and few of us enjoy eating alone. Yet, how often do ambulatory patients who spend time outside of their rooms go back to bed to eat as soon as the trays arrive?

We know of several hospitals where patients go to cafeterias or take their trays to day rooms. Often patients could be encouraged to at least sit in a chair at mealtime, or visit the patient next door. Providing a room with chairs and tables of a convenient height, so patients can eat together in a more pleasant environment, is done quite extensively in pediatric wards, but very seldom for adults in general wards.

We should allow and even encourage patients to dress for meals. Possibly, we could provide patients with clothing that is more appropriate for a cafeteria than nightgowns and bathrobes.

If patients wear their own frily nightgowns or eat in bed, they should have help in protecting their apparel. Tying a bib around a patient's neck and saying, "Now, don't be sloppy," is different from helping a patient place and cut the food. Patients have reported that rather than spill liquids, they just do not drink.

In other areas, we have seen metal trays with heavy dishes, whose weight and bulk are a burden to the aides who carry them and to the patients who hold the trays on their laps. Rather than attempt to pick up such heavy crockery, debilitated patients may give up in fatigue. Also, we have frequently heard patients objecting to plastic dishes, yet how often they are used in hospitals.

Terminology on selective menus must be understandable for most patients. Such terms as "julienne carrots" are meaningless to many.

TEACHING ABOUT FOODS

Food may be given as a reward or taken away as a punishment. Many times, nurses reward favorite patients for good behavior by giving them special food.

One thing that is common to all of us is our love for good food. There is a difference, however, between the scientific perspective of food and the so-called lay perspective. The health professional may regard food for patients as a means to improve health, almost in the category of drugs. They fear that if a patient does not get enough protein, hypoproteinemia may develop. On the other hand, patients usually regard food as something to satisfy hunger. They feel familiar with food and qualified to make judgments about it. These two perspectives can sometimes conflict.

Subtle thoughts and emotions that people associate with certain foods at times complicate and at times aid in both feeding and teaching patients. Patients may assume a food will not taste good if they know it is good for their health. Children associate vivid attributes with foods, for example, talking about "weak" peaches. Milk and cereal may symbolize baby food to a truck driver. Most nurses have heard persons who regard certain foods as "good for the blood."

FAMILIES AND VOLUNTEERS

To do the best possible job of feeding patients, we could utilize the patients' families and friends in more ways than we have thus far. Eating is a social time and a social tie, and yet, in many hospitals, visiting hours are not yet anywhere near meal hours. We should do more to enable patients' families to eat with patients. If this is to succeed, food must be priced so that patients' families can afford it. If a patient and his wife could have dinner together, the wife might learn more about what the patient should be eating. A relative might help to feed the patient. Also, family members may give us meaningful information about a patient's food habits that the patient himself is reluctant to give. If families are permitted to bring special foods from home, a patient may feel less anxiety. Food from home may be the so-called self-starter for a patient's appetite. Many times, this is the only way the patient's family can "do something" for the patient.

We can also make better use of women's auxiliaries and other volunteers. A volunteer from a certain culture may be able to talk with a patient about his food and help interpret to the staff. Volunteers can help feed patients or just sit and converse with patients while they eat.

Obviously, nurses cannot carry out all these suggestions by themselves. Other departments and personnel are involved. But nurses can choose what is appropriate in their own situations.

Certainly, patients will be better served if we remember that their responses to foods are conditioned by their own values.

What part does nutrition play in achieving optimum functioning?

How do you feel when you skip a meal or when you are too ill to eat? What changes do you expect to see in a child who is irritable because of mild hunger when he is given a meal? Would you expect the same change in an adult?

How might a nurse use some of the ideas presented in this article in helping a family care for a patient at home?

How might life style and cultural differences affect a persons on a prescribed diet? How can you find out a person's real life-style of eating?

List six ways to make eating in a hospital more enjoyable for a patient?

State two possible reasons that a patient may not be eating or taking fluids.

Why might a patient not be filling in a menu daily?

41.

Ulcer Patient: Emotional Emergency

Lynn R. Purintun
Louella Iles Nelson

The ulcer patient is difficult for himself and for you; why? What cues can you find as you read about Mr. B? Would you want to be his nurse?

"I've got no patience with someone like that—he comes in with a bleeding ulcer, then refuses to eat anything, including milk. Anybody who's a food faddist deserves an ulcer!"

"What a kook—he runs around opening all the windows and hanging his head out. He's so selfish, he doesn't even consider the other patients—opens the windows, disturbs them with his constant hollering. He won't do anything to help himself—won't take his feedings or his antacids. I just don't understand him."

The comments flew hot and heavy during the week following Mr. B.'s admission to the intensive care unit with the diagnosis of duodenal ulcer with hemorrhage (his hematocrit was 21 percent on admission). Mr. B. was a 67-year-old bachelor who had lived with his mother until her death four years before. He attributed the development of his ulcer to the fact that he had stopped drinking mineral water two months prior to his admission. Also, he announced frequently, he had been going to several special award dinners which consisted of "rich foods not good for you."

Slightly built, pale, and frail appearing, Mr. B. smiled nervously when he spoke and fingered the bedding, or swung his legs over the edge of the bed. He freely discussed his ideas about food and his belief that milk was harmful to adults and caused increased bleeding. His arguments against the regimen prescribed by his physicians indicated a considerable knowledge of nutrition and dietetics.

After a week in the intensive care unit, Mr. B. was not progressing. He seemed to be in constant motion, and his irritability rose daily, along with the frequency of his accusations and demands. Each disagreement with the staff seemed to precipitate another bleeding episode and his flat refusal again to take the prescribed food, medications, or treatments. Phenobarbital, morphine, and Vistaril were tried and then discontinued because they appeared to help only temporarily, and sometimes only increased his agitation.

The animosity between the staff and Mr. B. was close to the boiling point. A transfer to another ward was suggested, but there were no other beds available. Something had to be done. One physician described him as "agitated, rambunctious, and restless," and ordered that restraints be used if necessary.

The head nurse, after conferring with the surgical supervisor, asked the advice of a nursing instructor, and the two decided to schedule a conference for the following day to discuss Mr. B. To guide the staff in identifying the real problem and in gaining some insight into the underlying causes of Mr. B's behavior, they invited the mental health integrator from the college of nursing.

The next day, the nursing personnel on duty and the students met in the conference which was conducted by the mental health integrator. She began by asking the staff to tell her things about the patient which she could list on the blackboard.

This first step served two purposes. These statements allowed the nurses to express feelings which previously had not been dealt with openly. Second, listing the complaints enabled the group to deal with them one by one.

WHY THE ANGER?

The first statements about the patient were very angry, and as the staff watched the list grow, their negative feelings became increasingly apparent. As their awareness grew, they were able to begin asking why Mr. B. made them feel as they did and why he behaved as he did.

His Beliefs

One of the chief complaints involved Mr. B.'s belief in health foods, which he stated was his reason for ignoring the prescribed milk-antacid regimen.

The integrator pointed out that even though Mr. B.'s ideas about the harmfulness of milk appeared strange in our day and age, it was a belief held by many people for either religious or health reasons. His feeling about milk, she suggested, might be compared to our cultural attitude toward eating the heads or eyes of fish, which are considered delicacies by some groups.

His Demands

Second, the nursing staff felt they were never able to satisfy the patient's incessant demands. No matter what they did, he still became upset.

Again the integrator offered a brief explanation. She suggested that, as a government official, this man was probably accustomed to controlling situations. Therefore, it might be anticipated that he would have some trouble adjusting to a hospital routine in which he was expected to follow orders. She also reminded the group about studies which suggest that people with ulcers have an underlying dependency-independency conflict, so that they cannot accept the dependent role even temporarily because of the unresolved desire to be dependent, which they fear and deny.

His Abusiveness

The third major complaint about Mr. B. was his general attitude of uncoopera- tiveness, and the unpleasant way he responded to nursing personnel, to the point of using abusive language. It was noted, however, that Mr. B. was generally more cooperative with the nursing students than he was with the staff.

The integrator asked the staff what anxieties they thought this man might have in relation to his current hospitalization, and the staff listed several: anxieties about cancer, dying, helplessness, incapacity, and the conflict between his food practices and the medical orders.

With the preceding information on the blackboard, the nurses were asked to think about the reasons for the present situation. The participants began to look critically at their own feelings. One nurse stated that feelings might be interfering with the rational side of behavior for everyone involved. The nurses, thinking that they were right, had told Mr. B. what to do without considering what he wanted to do or providing him with an adequate explanation. Although he reacted negatively, they had persisted in the same approaches.

"WHAT ARE WE GIVING HIM?"

Inattention

Mr. B., who complained about lack of attention, actually was in this situation receiving less attention than the other patients because he was in the intensive care unit, where everyone else had just had surgery. In addition, the amount of time voluntarily spent with him decreased as he became more unpleasant. The nurses decided they had not considered how much attention *he thought* he needed.

Disapproval

The staff also added to the list of reasons their expectations of and attitudes toward the patient. Some said they had expected him to be unpleasant, after learning he was a government official.

They also decided that, after reading on his history that he was a food faddist, they had blamed him for creating his own problems without any real attempt to find out what the faddism involved.

Finally, Mr. B. talked openly of an affair he was having with a married woman, which further increased the nurses' feelings of dislike and disapproval.

The staff decided, therefore, that a vicious circle had started with Mr. B. They had reacted with avoidance, authoritarianism, and threats in response to Mr. B.'s animosity. These reactions, in turn, only increased his undesirable behavior.

Defensiveness
Looking back at this response to the patient, staff members noted that they had taken personally all of the statements made by the patient, rather than looking at them as his attempts to express his feelings of frustration and anxiety. The integrator pointed out that, while everyone wishes to be liked, in order to carry out adequate patient care, it is advantageous to look beyond one's personal reactions in order to get at the reasons for negative behavior?

She suggested that the patient resorted to name-calling and placing blame on the nurses to make them feel inadequate so that he would feel adequate in comparison, and not quite so dependent on them. She further explained that, when the nurses responded by acting even more restrictive and authoritarian, Mr. B.'s anxieties were increased. The students who were less authoritarian, therefore had fewer difficulties with Mr. B.

"WHAT SHALL WE TRY"

Beginning with the first complaint, about Mr. B.'s attitude toward food, the staff went down the list, making concrete suggestions.

The Food Problem
Each would try to understand Mr. B.'s beliefs and their influence on his behavior, attempting to increase her background information in an effort to understand and accept rather than to make judgments on first impressions or limited information.

The staff would work to separate their expectations of the way people should act from the way Mr. B. actually behaved. They realized they could not impose their values on him any more than they expected Mr. B. to impose his on them.

One of the dieticians would be asked to work with the patient in formulating a diet that was compatible both with his food beliefs and the medical requirements.

His Need for Control

After recognizing the patient's demands as an expression of his need to exert control and independence, the staff agreed that he would be given an explanation of all procedures carried out for him so that he would have the feeling of *at least* knowing what was being done for him and why.

Mr. B. would be allowed to participate in his own care as much as he wished and was physically and emotionally able. He would be offered opportunities to make as many decisions for himself as were realistic.

Before leaving Mr. B.'s bedside, the nurse would tell him when she planned to return, and that he could call before then if he had any requests. The staff would answer his requests promptly and stop by his bed at regular intervals to see if he needed anything before he had to call. The staff felt this was especially important since Mr. B. seemed to have many anxieties about the possibility of surgery. (This was the approach with which the nursing students had had success.)

Reducing His Fears

Once they viewed Mr. B.'s uncooperativeness as an expression of his anxieties, the staff decided they needed to spend time getting to know him better as a person. They would allow him opportunities to talk about the things that might be bothering him, encourage him to ask questions about areas in which he wanted more information, and attempt to answer these questions to his satisfaction.

The staff agreed that they should let Mr. B. know that they did care for him and were concerned about what happened to him. They would attempt to accomplish this by listening, by respecting his wishes and preferences whenever possible, and by spending time with him other than when he called for their help.

Prevention

The final suggestion made by the staff was that they should make further attempts to recognize the role their own feelings play in patient care, and plan to set aside time to talk about and deal with these feelings before they interfered with patient welfare.

VICIOUS CIRCLE BROKEN

One nursing student seemed particularly interested in the welfare of this patient. As soon as she left the conference, she returned to Mr. B. and spent time listening and talking to him, answering his questions, and teaching him about his illness. At the end of the conversation, Mr. B. agreed to sign the operative permit—something he had refused to do in three days—for a gastrectomy and vagotomy.

Surgery was scheduled for the next day and the nursing student was there early that morning to give Mr. B. his preoperative medications and to offer support. She followed him to surgery, the recovery room, and back to the intensive care unit, caring for him on his first postoperative day as well. Mr. B. had come through surgery without event and responded positively to the care and concern shown him by this student and other staff.

Subsequent conferences about Mr. B. were conducted by the head nurse with staff members who had not been present for the original conference. It appeared that the information exchanged at the first conference was relayed accurately, for the other staff members also made an effort to use the suggestions.

When the nursing students and their instructor returned to the hospital the following week after a four-day absence, they were pleasantly surprised to learn that in this time Mr. B. had improved sufficiently to have been transferred from the intensive care unit to floor care. For the first time since his admission, he appeared friendly and relaxed, smiled at the staff, and engaged in conversation. The staff reported that the name-calling and incessant demands had virtually ceased. Mr. B. had talked with the dietitian, and together they had been able to develop a diet compatible with his food beliefs without seriously compromising the medical regimen. He was now taking some milk products and offered no resistance to medications.

During the remainder of Mr. B.'s hospitalization, the nursing student spent considerable time talking to him, listening to his ideas about food, and reading some of the literature about food that he had brought to the hospital. In return, Mr. B. listened to the student's explanations of anatomy and physiology, the surgery he had recently undergone, and the rationale for his therapy. In addition, she discussed with him his plans for the future and helped him set realistic short-term and long-range goals.

Information obtained through this work with Mr. B. was shared with all nursing personnel via follow-up evaluative conferences and current notations on the Kardex.

As Mr. B. began to react positively to the change in the approaches of the nursing staff, they, in turn, became even more involved in meeting Mr. B.'s nursing needs. This genuine interest and concern was communicated to Mr. B., who in response began to trust them. As he did so, many of his fears appeared to decrease and, consequently, most of the behavior which the staff had found objectionable ceased.

What does his comment that "milk is harmful to adults and caused increased bleeding" indicate to you about his acceptance of his problem?

What was the purpose of listing on the blackboard the observations made by the staff during the conference?

List the integrator's interpretation of each problem. What other interpretation had you thought of? Why do you agree or disagree? Who in your hospital acts as an integrator? What title is used?

Why did students have less difficulty with Mr. B?

What approach did the staff take in order to *prevent* further problems?

Write down the steps you can identify of Mr. B.'s "vicious circle" and indicate how it was broken.

Visualize yourself as the team leader and holding a team conference about this patient. How would you have started the discussion and helped the group arrive at some solutions?

42.
Preoperative Anxiety

Doris L. Carnevali

The following article summarizes studies done with preoperative patients to find out if patient needs are recognized in the clinical setting. What are the major preoperative concerns? List them here.

Check those that you have observed as you cared for patients before surgery.

The current concept of professional nursing is that nursing actions are deliberative, based on knowledgeable interpretation of patient data. But the effectiveness of these nursing actions depends upon how accurately the nurse perceives the patient's response to his illness, to the experience of being ill, and to the nursing intervention.

The preoperative period is normally a stressful, anxiety-ridden time in a patient's life when the activities of the nurse may be particularly important in providing support and comfort as well as the routine physical ministrations required. If we believe that appropriate nursing actions are based on perceived patient needs, we need to find out how well, within the reality of the clinical setting, we recognize these needs.

Three studies have been undertaken in attempts to find some answers to this question.

Contacts between the nurse investigators and the patients consisted of brief structured interviews. Twelve to 15 open-ended questions were asked in the first two studies. The third used a rating scale with planned probes. Most of the patients seemed willing — even eager — to talk, despite the presence of a tape recorder. Even though the interviewers were limited to neutral responses in this interaction, patients later indicated that having had an opportunity to talk about their feelings had made them more comfortable. This seems to indicate that many patients, given an opportunity, would willingly share their perceptions and expectations with their nurses. One investigator was concerned that she might increase patients' fears by exploring them preoperatively. But experience with 71 patients in the last two studies proved this concern unfounded.

The sources of concern reported by patients in the three studies fell into categories previously reported in the literature. Pain and discomfort were mentioned most frequently. Almost as many were worried about not knowing what to expect. A special and recurrent area of this, "unknown" category was the fear that they had not been told "the whole truth" about diagnoses.

Disturbance over changes in the body resulting from surgery was sometimes found to be related to the extensiveness of the surgery, but this appeared to be a deep concern in many patients in whom it might not have been anticipated. Abhorrence of being "cut," or comments such as, "I just won't feel the same even if nobody ever sees the incision" demonstrate that any surgical patient may feel his body image threatened.

Many patients feared separation: they worried about how their families or spouses were getting along.

Fear due to previous surgical experience was related not only to the patients' own experiences but to those of family and friends as well. And medical television programs, currently available to millions, supply additional vicarious experiences which influence attitudes.

Some patients in each study group voiced a fear of death — eight out 11 in the second study. Six of these 11 patients had tentative or positive diagnoses of malignancy. One patient in the first study who knew death was imminent without surgery, and that it was a real possibility during surgery, read of the death of another patient following similar surgery in the same hospital. She said, after reading it, "I die right with him."

Disruption of life plans was found to be related to the patients' recreational as well as occupational life. In fact, candidates for "more serious" surgery were more concerned about disruption of recreational life than of occupational life.

Patients in all the studies were concerned about losing control, many speaking of it in terms of the anesthesia.

Finances were reported as a problem by patients in private hospitals, but not in the federal hospital where the third study was done.

Only two patients indicated that they had no concerns. One was an elderly gentleman with parkinsonism. The second said that he had waited too long for treatment and that he would have to take things as they came; he seemed calmly fatalistic.

The first two studies revealed what nurses thought the 21 patients were concerned about preoperatively.

Nurses did not seem to be aware that so many patients were concerned about pain and discomfort. On the other hand, they tended to be quite accurate in perceiving patient worry about the unknown.

DOES TIME MATTER?

The first study seemed to show that nurses were much more aware of the concerns of patients who were in the hospital more than 24 hours before surgery than they were of those who were there less than a day.

TESTING PATIENTS' ANSWERS

Another incidental finding of these studies was that the indirect question was an effective means of verifying patients' responses. The patient was asked to put himself in the place of the nurse, and then to indicate what he would expect someone else facing similar surgery would be concerned about. Some patients verified what they had already said: "Well, I guess he'd worry about the same things I was worried about." On the other hand, there was a patient facing brain surgery who had talked about her concern for her daughter's well-being, her desire to have her muscle spasm relieved, and her eagerness to have surgery, despite the cautions of friends. When she was asked what another patient might worry about, she said, "Oh, she'd be worried about whether she'd be blind, whether she could talk, and whether her personality would change. Those are the things you are so afraid of that you don't ask, for fear you'll find out what you don't want to hear." If her nurses had perceived the question she was really asking when she said, "Will I be able to see my husband after surgery?" they might have spared her some anxiety, since blindness was not a complication associated with her surgical procedure.

DECREASING DISTRESS

What did nurses do to alleviate patients' preoperative distress? Determining congruence between patients' and nurses' perceptions in this area was more difficult, since each was likely to view the same action quite differently. One nurse said, "As I got him ready I told him why I did these things. I told him that after he came back we'd want him to cough, move about and take deep breaths." Another nurse caring for the same patient said, "I stood by his bed for a while and talked to him (they were waiting for the patient to leave for surgery). I told him we would be waiting for him to come back." The patient said, "I've never seen nicer people."

Another nurse said, "There were no physical things to do for him on the night before surgery, so I popped in occasionally when I was at that end of the ward — just so he wouldn't feel neglected." This patient said, "They somehow create the feeling that, well, here we are one great big happy family." Questioned further, he added, "It's more of an attitude than what's said."

Usually, the nurse thought she imparted knowledge, while the patient said she offered friendliness and interest in him as a person. Thus, when the responses were tabulated, patients' observations on how the nurses relieved preoperative concerns, in order of descending frequency, were: reassurance and friendliness, nursing skill and competence, concern and interest in the patient, willingness to listen, and, lowest on the list, decreasing the unknown. No patient cited diversion as alleviating preoperative uneasiness.

Nurses, however, commented most frequently on decreasing the unknown (in 19 out of 21 patients); next, on reassuring the patient that he had been wise in deciding to have treatment and that he had competent medical care; third, listening to the patient; then, showing concern and acceptance; conveying a feeling of security through nursing competence; and, least frequently, diversion.

One or more nurses stated they had done nothing to decrease preoperative uneasiness in two patients. One of these patients also said the nurses had done nothing, but the second identified many nursing actions which she had found supportive.

INCREASING DISTRESS

A few patients reported nursing actions which actually increased their preoperative distress. One felt that the insertion of a nasogastric tube before she was awake enough to cooperate properly had been more than necessarily traumatic. Another patient was taken into a semilighted surgical suite to wait as nurses prepared the operating room. The nurses were disagreeing as to whether the room was large enough to do the particular procedure. The patient remembered wondering whether they would continue to disagree during the operation, and feared this might affect the outcome of his surgery.

SUMMARY

As nurses, we are challenged to come to know each patient within a limited time; and, to the extent it is possible, to perceive his needs and act to meet them, attempting to alleviate or prevent his distress. The constant flow of surgical patients through our wards offers us daily opportunity to perfect our skill — in observing with greater acuity and in acting effectively.

List the fears or concerns stated in the article that you had previously been unaware of. What cues would you look or listen for while talking with preoperative patients?

What was the effect on the fears when these were explored postoperatively?

Think about and then try the indirect approach to see how a patient might think another person would feel facing a certain surgical procedure.

PART V

SOME INTENSIVE SKILLS

The articles in this section require a basic knowledge of nursing care. Each demonstrates an acute health problem where the medical team must act quickly and correctly to reverse the damage being done to the body.

These situations take place in emergency rooms, intensive care and coronary care units, and in acute medical and surgical units. Each challenges the nurse to apply skillful nursing care.

43.

The New E.R. Nursing — Is It For You?

Rhea Felknor

The following two articles provide a clear picture of the knowledge and skills needed to care for emergency victims. Evaluate yourself as you read them and find out where your own strengths and weaknesses lie. Do you like change? Are your impatient with routine? Read on – E. R. Nursing may be for you!

In the last three years emergency department procedures have increasingly come to be looked upon as a medical specialty. Today there are three basic types of emergency departments, and the nurse's responsibilities can vary considerably, depending upon the type to which she is assigned:

1. *The major emergency department* is a 24-hour comprehensive facility, fully equipped and staffed to render the most complex and comprehensive emergency care. Only a few of the larger hospitals in a region have one. Here the most advanced emergency surgical and medical procedures are routinely performed, including cardiac surgery, the treatment of severe head wounds, major plastic surgery. The facility is staffed 24 hours a day by a team of physicians, nurses, and support personnel who frequently find themselves working simultaneously on a patient with multiple injuries.

2. *The limited emergency department* has a resident physician available on call. Physicians covering most specialties are available in the community. Triage is usually handled by the nurse. This E.R. can deal with most life-threatening emergencies, but doesn't have highly specialized resuscitative and surgical equipment. However, a blood bank, laboratory, X-ray, and other diagnostic facilities are constantly available.

From "The New E. R. Nursing–Is It For You?" by Rhea Felknor, published in the November 1970 issue of R.N. *Copyright © 1970 by* R.N. *Reproduced, with permission, from* R.N.

3. *The provisional emergency unit* in small hospitals or industrial plants depends upon the R.N. to make the initial assessment of the victim's condition and telephone a doctor — who, however, may not be able to arrive for some time. The nurse treats minor injuries and provides emergency resuscitation, knows how to control external blood loss, maintain an airway, and perform external cardiopulmonary resuscitation. All but minor injuries are taken to nearby larger emergency facilities.

In a big city (where all three types of E.R.s may exist), up to 90 per cent of the people who come to the department may be using it simply as a doctor's office.

They come at all hours of the day and night — a trend particularly evident since the start of Medicare and Medicaid. The "new" E.R. nurse has to be adept at handling them. Otherwise they could tie up so much of her time that she wouldn't be able to take care of the actual emergencies.

"Many of these people, particularly the poor, have been made aware that good health care is a right," says Dr. Robert J. Freeark of Chicago. "They are no longer content to go to a clinic, wait all day, and then be told to come back tomorrow because the clinic closes at 5."

Dr. Freeark foresees the day when metropolitan hospitals will provide extensive clinic facilities near the emergency department, solely to diagnose and treat ambulatory patients who come with complaints about such things as vague abdominal pains, weight loss, and a cough.

Is E.R. nursing for you? Well, here's what it requires of the nurse today, in the view of the experts:

1. *Knowledge.* Good nursing practice in the E.R. involves actions that are considered the practice of medicine when they are performed in other than an emergency situation. "If the R.N. is to render effective care in an emergency room, she needs some post-graduate education," says Dr. George T. Anast, the orthopedic surgeon who is a member of the American College of Surgeons' famed Chicago Committee on Trauma.

Knowledgeable experts say 20 per cent of the deaths due to auto accidents and cardiac arrests could be prevented if E.R. personnel were better trained.

What must the emergency care nurse know?

"Airway defects kill most of the people who die in highway accidents," says Dr. J.D. Farrington. "So the nurse has to know how to establish and maintain an airway."

Dr. Farrington believes E.R. nurses should also know how to provide oxygen inhalation and intermittent positive-pressure ventilation, perform cardiopulmonary resuscitation, control accessible bleeding, administer I.V. fluids, give care to patients who have been poisoned, immobilize fractures, perform emergency deliveries, and manage unruly patients. A number of authorities also want her to know how to read ECGs for basic patterns, and be prepared to defibrillate electrically.

"The emergency department nurse needs more training not only because of the types of cases she sees, but because many of her patients are in shock or emotionally upset," says Judith C. Kelleher, R.N., head E.R. nurse at the 150-bed Downey (Calif.) Community Hospital.

One way to provide emotional support and head off outbursts is to keep the patient and his family informed of what is going on, she says. "The nurse can't be smug in answering their questions," she emphasizes. "We try to keep the family members involved as much as possible – we offer them a cup of coffee, invite them to watch television, and do other things to show that we really care.

"In the event of a death or an emotional upset, we can take the family into our coffee room for privacy, and call our chaplain or their own minister, rabbi, or priest and our nurses are never too busy to offer a shoulder to cry on."

Dr. Anast, head of the Ravenswood Trauma Unit, has trained his nurses to splint fractures and put on castlike devices by themselves.

In a medium-sized E.R. like that of the St. Louis (Mo.) County Hospital, nurses may do such things as assess the patient's condition, assign priorities for treatment, treat superficial problems themselves, and call the doctor for others.

For example, when a child with a deep laceration came to the E.R. recently, Linda Wendell, R.N., cleaned the child's laceration, prepared the suturing setup, gave the tetanus injection the doctor had ordered, and recorded all the things she had done. When the doctor came, he could tell the patient's status by glancing at the card. He sutured the wound, and Mrs. Wendell then applied the dressing and cleaned up.

Most emergency department nurses don't consider it beneath their dignity to do needed "scut work."

"We work together to get the job done," Mrs. Wendell says.

The good E.R. nurse needs to know not only how to do her job but also how to keep her cool. Dr. Freeark lists "imperturbability" as her most desirable trait. "She's got to be all things to all people," he explains. "She's got to handle the family and the police and the politician and the thief and the drug addict, and handle them all with compassion as well as efficiency. A hospital's reputation in the community is to an increasing extent being determined by the kind of emergency department care it gives – and this depends in large measure upon the attitude and performance of the nurse."

2. *Initiative.* "The emergency department nurse has to be interested and willing to act," says Dr. Farrington. "She has to develop an inquiring mind, not just skills. On her own, while waiting for the physician, she must be willing to stop accessible bleeding, correct any airway defect, institute pulmonary resuscitation, start an infusion, treat for shock, and do anything else required by life-threatening problems."

Dr. Freeark believes many E.R. nurses should be more aggressive than they have been in taking responsibility. He suggests triage as a field in which nurses could be more active.

"R.N.s can do it, and do it well," he says. "I have found over the years that nurses are better than interns in making decisions on who should stay in the E.R. and who should go home. They perceive many things that need to be done that most doctors aren't aware of, and go ahead and do them. The R.N. is more aware of psychological and social needs, for example, and in other ways has more compassion for her patients."

As nursing licensure acts are broadened to permit nurses to do more procedures, many doctors foresee increasing prestige for the E.R. nurse.

"And prestige won't be the only thing she'll get," says Dr. Anast. "No one should expect a nurse to practice medicine at a nurse's salary. The more a nurse does, the more responsibility she takes, the more pay she should get."

3. *Skill.* In Buffalo, Mrs. Dorr sees to it that each nurse who will be working in the E.R. is first rotated through the O.R., I.C.U., and C.C.U. The R.N. works with the people in anesthesia until the anesthesiologist says she is ready to resuscitate, and with the people in cardiology until the cardiologist believes she is ready to perform ECGs. E.R. nurses often go out with the ambulance to administer aid to cardiac or stroke victims.

Knowledge, initiative, skill — three characteristics of the good E.R. nurse. There is a fourth: spunk.

"It takes a special kind of person to work in the emergency facility, a nurse with real spirit," says Dr. Heck. One veteran nurse attributes her gray hairs to the decisions she was not afraid to make "during the 15 minutes before the doctor arrived." Anita Dorr won't hire a nurse for the E.R. unless she is convinced she has "spirit."

"She has to have the courage of her convictions," explains Mrs. Dorr. "Emergency room nursing takes a high-strung individual, someone who is dissatisfied with routine, someone who likes change."

Resuscitation equipment
the R.R. nurse uses

There are no nationally accepted standards for equipping emergency services, so each E.R. varies. The following is the resuscitation equipment list recommended at the Airlie Conference on Emergency Medical Services held in Warrenton, Va., in early 1969 under sponsorship of the American College of Surgeons and the American Academy of Orthopaedic Surgeons:

1. Oxygen, either via wall outlets or mobile carts, with flow meters and delivery tubes.
2. Bag-valve-mask units with oxygen reservoir tubings.
3. Oropharyngeal and nasopharyngeal airways of various sizes.
4. Suction equipment.
5. Tracheal intubation kit, including equipment for gastric intubation.
6. Emergency drug kit.
7. Injection/infusion kit, including needles, syringes, catheters, stopcocks, venotubes, administration sets, blood substitutes (e.g., dextran 75 or 5 per cent albumin, dextran 40, isotonic saline solution, dextrose in Ringer's solution) blood (type O, Rh negative—refrigerated), blood warmer, equipment for infusion under pressure.
8. Venous cutdown tray.
9. Separate crash cart with electrocardioscope (needle and disk electrodes), external/internal defibrillator with appropriate electrodes and battery-powered pacemaker.
10. Electrocardiograph.
11. Tracheostomy tray.
12. Thoracotomy tray for open-chest cardiac resuscitation.
13. Pleural drainage tray (with trocars and catheters of various sizes; Heimlich valves or water-seal drainage bottles).
14. Equipment for central venous pressure catheterization.
15. Equipment for arterial puncture and catheterization.
16. Tray for nerve blocks and local anesthesia.
17. Ventilating bronchoscope (all sizes, available in hospital).
18. Mechanical ventilator capable of producing assisted and controlled intermittent positive pressure ventilation with 100 per cent oxygen, drug aerosols, and heated mist, with airway pressures and tidal volumes readable.

All equipment should be suitable for adults, children, and infants. Respiratory equipment must have standard 15 mm. tracheal tube and 22 mm. mask connectors.

44.

Let's Have More E.R. Courses!

Etta M. Rosenthal

It's late at night. You're a nurse in a small-town hospital, alone in the emergency room. The nearest doctor is 50 miles away.

Suddenly the door flies open and a man staggers in. He is bleeding from multiple head and chest wounds, and his right arm hangs limply at his side. Just before he falls to the floor, unconscious, he gasps that he has been in an auto accident and that his wife is still trapped inside the car.

What is the first thing you do?

Or, you're a nurse on duty in a big-city E.R. A frantic mother runs in with her crying baby. He has burns over 40 per cent of his body. Just as you're placing the child on the gurney, a heart attack victim is brought into the room. His color is poor, his chest isn't moving, and you can't get a radial pulse. The orderly just left for the I.C.U., and the nurse's aide is at lunch. What do you do — first?

Unusual situations? Anyone working in E.R. will tell you they're not! And they bring up some uncomfortable questions: How many nurses — and how many doctors — are adequately trained to recognize priority symptoms? And how many emergency rooms are adequately equipped to handle a wide variety of casualties at a moment's notice?

For some time the American Academy of Orthopaedic Surgeons, the American College of Surgeons, and the Chicago Trauma Committee have recognized that the prognosis of bone and other injuries is dependent on proper primary treatment, since wrong handling can result in irreversible damage. During the last five years both organizations have sponsored post-graduate courses for emergency room nurses, covering subjects you can't get in other nursing studies. I recently attended such a course in San Diego.

Since blocked ventilation is such a common problem in emergencies, opening the airway and keeping it open received major emphasis.

"Remember, if your patient stops breathing suddenly, you've got only four minutes," warned Dr. Stephen Murphy. "If you don't act at once, there will be irreversible brain damage. So survey your patient first, and then move!

"Learn to use your stethoscope to determine if your patient needs suctioning — you *must* open that airway! It can be filled with gravel, pus, blood, even somebody's severed ear. To determine if it is blocked, put your hand over his mouth and feel the air and listen, by putting your ear near his mouth. If obstruction is evident, turn the patient on his side to drain his mouth. Have the suction available and always hooked up, ready to use. You must suction the pharynx, but don't do it until any foreign bodies are removed. A metal spoon (never plastic!) is better than your fingers to scoop out the mouth. Watch out for dental prostheses — they're expensive to replace, and the patient could swallow them. Tonsil suctions are often more difficult to use than plastic catheters. Keep your biggest catheters on hand. Suction *after* the food and debris are removed, otherwise they'll clog the catheter.

"Be sure the suction machines are properly hooked up, with a large catheter at the ready, and have a plastic Levin tube passed down the patient's nose. Plastic is preferred because it is less likely to kink. Although you have to work fast, be sure O_2 is not going into the patient's stomach — it could blow the stomach out. The introduction of even a small amount of air or O_2 may cause the stomach contents to be regurgitated, and this may result in aspiration. Patients have been known to die a week later from aspirated vomitus."

Dr. Murphy's instructions on placing an airway tube are equally pungent: "Keep the patient's chin up and his neck back, so that his head is extended. Select a proper size airway — it doesn't matter if it sticks out of his mouth. If his face is injured, use a soft nasal airway. Match the airway up on the outside of his face, use a lubricant such as Xylocaine — lubrication with water is a waste of time. You must look at the chest; if it's not moving, you're not ventilating!"

What about mouth-to-mouth resuscitation?

"Learn to use the resuscitation equipment so you don't have to use your mouth — that's an unnecessary hazard for you, and the airway is much more efficient," Dr. Murphy said. "In placing the airway, feed it back with the curved portion down, so that when you get it in, it lies behind the tongue. Don't force it if it won't go any further."

He gave explicit instructions on what to do when you can't feel a pulse on the patient anywhere. "You *must* start artificial circulation," he said. "In my opinion, the effectiveness of chest-compressing machines is unproven. So do the procedures manually."

The next day the technics and pitfalls of endotracheal intubation were explored. Dr. Murphy feels the E.R. nurse should be thoroughly trained in this procedure, and suggested that it be practiced on D.O.A. at autopsies, and on patients without hope. He also urged that a separate tray be kept in the E.R. for children, with Miller blades available in infant and preemie sizes, and that disposable airways and tubes be utilized whenever possible.

"Keep drugs off the resuscitation trays!" he emphasized. "Time is of the essence, and we need quick, easy access to the resuscitation equipment."

All of the doctors emphasized that nurses should know how to handle all equipment used in the E.R., and should be given more latitude in administering treatment and performing tests, such as ECGs.

Insulin shock, diabetic coma, electrolyte abnormalities, and dental emergencies were dealt with in detail.

"If you suspect that teeth are missing, be sure the doctor checks through X-rays before suturing — especially where there is a split mandible," he said. Slides were shown, indicating what happens when teeth and bone fragments become embedded and are overlooked, resulting in infection, pain, and subsequent surgery.

"Prognosis depends upon initial care!" a plastic surgeon, Dr. Lawrence T. Moore, told us. "Above everything else, please follow meticulous wound-cleansing procedures in taking care of facial injuries. Remove the dirt and the blood clots! However, facial wounds do not have precedence, and their care should not compromise the patient. They can be treated even as long as 24 hours after the accident because of the good blood supply the face normally has."

He prefers using a 1 per cent Xylocaine solution with a dilution of 1:1,000 epinephrine to infiltrate around the edges of wounds.

"Save all the pieces!" he pleaded. "We can later throw away what we don't need.

"Begin closure at key points, especially at lip borders and at eyelids, because edema starts rapidly there. Eliminate dead space. You know, of course, never to shave an eyebrow. Whenever possible, prep a possible donor site ahead of time. In debridement, be intelligent and conservative. And don't allow wound edges to curl under."

If any of the nurses had never seen a hyphema (hemorrhage into the anterior chamber of the eye — behind the cornea and in front of the lens) they will surely recognize one in the future after seeing the slides shown by Dr. George L. Tabor, an ophthalmologist. The slides indicated the disastrously quick, progressive damage caused when this symptom is ignored. He urged nurses to watch for this warning sign, and point it out to examining physicians in the event they did not notice it. Such patients require immediate bed rest, eye patches, and the care of an opthalmologist as soon as possible.

Dr. Tabor reviewed the effects of both acid and alkali eye burns. His advice in such cases: Don't bother to look for a neutralizing agent, but get to the eye fast and wash, wash, wash! He also emphasized that when a patient has foreign bodies superficially lodged in the cornea and it's apparent that there will be a 24-hour wait for a physician, the E.R. nurse should remove them.

The treatment of drug addicts brought many questions.

"If you have to confront addicts while alone, remember that they are not usually a threat," he told us. "That is, all except the amphetamine users — these people *are* potentially dangerous."

And there you have it — some highlights from the San Diego course for E.R. nurses. Those of us who took part will never forget the pleasure of meeting and talking to other E.R. nurses with similar problems. Somehow, we all feel more assured, more confident that we'll be able to handle the next patient who walks or is carried through the doors of our E.R., regardless of the challenge presented.

How do you know nasal oxygen is not entering a patient's stomach? One observation will tell you. If you don't know it now, look it up because this one skill that is not reserved for emergencies.

How do you fit a bag and mask to a face to avoid leaking? What equipment would you use to wash out an eye that had been injured with an acid or alkali? How long would it take to get the irrigation started? What solution would you use if a physician were not present?

Which of the items listed on page 287 can you operate? How could you learn to operate the rest?

45.

Emergency Care for Near-Drowning Victims

Bernice L. Shaw

You may wish to review articles 36 and 37 on fluids and electrolytes prior to or following your reading of this article. Metabolic acidosis can be a killer. When can it occur?

What happens to the fluid that enters a persons lungs during drowning? Is it absorbed into the body?

It was a gorgeous July Sunday. The emergency room at our East Coast hospital had been a madhouse since about 10:30 A.M. Then around 3 P.M. a police car arrived hurriedly and discharged its two passengers: a distraught father and his unresponsive 11-year-old son — victim of near-drowning.

Emergency measures were instituted immediately, and while the resident worked quickly over the boy, he calmly asked the father if the boy had been swimming in fresh or salt water. The father's quick reply betrayed his anxiety and impatience: "What difference does it make, Doc? His lungs are full of it!"

Ask a silly question, get a silly answer, I thought. Then, as if he'd heard me, the resident slowly smiled. "Treatmentwise, it makes little difference. But the sequence of physiological change does vary, so it would be helpful for me to know the type of water involved."

Salt water proved to be the culprit in this case, and we set to work. Our treatment was directed at combating the four main problems associated with near-drowning: impaired ventilation, metabolic acidosis, hypoxemia, and circulatory embarrassment. By the time the family's attending physician had arrived in the E.R., the patient's condition had improved remarkably. Nonetheless, the boy was not discharged but was admitted for 48 hours of observation. Grateful but disappointed, the family consoled themselves with the adage: Better safe than sorry.

* * *

The hospital nurse who has not given care to a near-drowning victim for some time may ask: Have new treatment methods been developed? Why are these patients often held for observation? In the past, those who recovered quickly were discharged directly from the E.R.

There is no "new" treatment as such, I found by studying the recent literature. But the treatment of metabolic acidosis is now being heralded by an increasing number of physicians as the first priority after a clear airway has been established. One or two ampules of sodium bicarbonate (44.6 mEq./ampule) are given initially, sometimes at the drowning scene or in the ambulance. Thereafter, blood gas analyses are used to determine future doses. If a patient's condition doesn't appear too serious, administration may be delayed until the arterial blood gas analysis is available at the hospital. When indicated and used, sodium bicarbonate can bring positive results in an amazingly short time.

Ventilation support is, of course, the priority at the drowning scene. It is started as soon as possible — with no time wasted trying to empty the victim's lungs. If the victim is breathing on his own, he is watched to see if some type of mechanical support such as I.P.P.B. is needed. Mouth-to-mouth resuscitation has proved an effective way to support ventilation until mechanical means are available. Endotracheal intubation is sometimes necessary, but tracheostomy rarely is.

Hypoxemia is treated with 100 per cent oxygen by mask or endotracheal tube as soon as possible, preferably at the drowning site. It is administered until the patient's arterial oxygen tensions can be maintained satisfactorily by his own revived breathing.

The amount of circulatory assistance given is determined by the need. If blood pressure and pulse are very weak or absent, external cardiac massage is usually indicated. Fluid therapy, administered via I.V. cutdown, is sometimes necessary. Oxygen and cardiotonics may also be employed.

What about the physiological effects of fresh water or salt water in the lungs? Either may be serious enough to require at least 48 hours of hospital observation after the patient's initial recovery.

When a person's lungs fill with fresh water, the water is absorbed very rapidly by the circulating blood. The blood volume can double in as little as two minutes, and from there on things can snowball. Massive destruction of red blood cells, severe electrolyte loss, and dilution of plasma proteins can result from hemodilution and osmotic loss into remaining lung fluids. Hypoxia can then trigger ventricular fibrillation and death. Or the hypervolemia can cause massive pulmonary edema and cardiac failure.

When sea water (a hypertonic solution of mixed salts) fills the lungs, the electrolytes therein rush into the blood. Blood sodium levels soar and pull circulating fluid into the lungs. Potassium levels drop, cardiac output is impaired, alveolar membranes deteriorate, and pulmonary edema, shock, and death can follow.

Fortunately, the metabolic acidosis resulting from either type of drowning is relatively easy to control provided measures can be taken promptly. As we've seen, it helps the doctor to know which type of physiological response he is dealing with.

Why does metabolic acidosis occur when respirations cease?

How does it affect the action of other life saving drugs being administered?

Why are sodium lactate and sodium bicarbonate administered, and how are each given?

List the symptoms that would make you suspect metabolic acidosis?

46.

Three Days with Mrs. M.

Carol R. Baxter

Patients with serious illness and impending surgery must face the possibility of residual damage or impairment and/or death. As you read this article, look for cues from the patient as this nurse observes, listens, and talks with her. What cues do the family members give?

As I entered the radioisotope department, Mrs. M. was sitting in the one chair in the waiting room. She was middle-aged, graying, pleasingly plump, and maternal. The only hint of anxiety was her nervous gesture of wringing her hands occasionally. The radiologist, who followed me into the room, explained the brain scan procedure to her. She seemed to accept the explanation stoically and asked no questions. This was my introduction to Mrs. M., and I marveled at the strength and fortitude she mustered as she faced this crisis in her life.

The first day I took care of Mrs. M., but before I even had a chance to look at her chart, one of the nursing students told me that Mrs. M. appeared anxious and upset and was crying. Mrs. M. was afraid, the student told me, that her hospitalization might precipitate a heart attack in her husband who had had two heart attacks in five years.

By the time I approached Mrs. M., she had stopped crying and had regained her composure. However, she still sat on the edge of her bed and appeared to be apprehensive; she continually played with her handkerchief and glanced furtively around the ward. I proceeded to explain that I was a student in the university, and would be caring for her. She responded by saying that it was too bad that I had to be "stuck" with her. When I told her that I had selected her to care for, she said that she would try to be a "good" patient.

At this point in the conversation, her eyes filled with tears, and she voiced her fears concerning her husband's health. She attempted to reassure me that she was unafraid of the surgery for herself. But, in the next breath, she informed me of her sleepless and restless night. She explained that she felt as though she was on the brink of exhaustion, but could not even lie down.

She repeatedly mentioned concern for her husband. Then, she branched out to include her daughter and recently married son. Since I felt there was an underlying problem which was not being aired, I responded to one of her repeated remarks about her husband by suggesting that it is important to be concerned about our families, but sometimes we are justified in being concerned for ourselves.

At this, Mrs. M began to cry. I waited. After a few minutes, she revealed her fear of the surgery, of the mutilating potential it held, and of the possibility that she would not survive. She spoke for 15 minutes. I just listened.

In this communication, I attempted to alleviate Mrs. M.'s discomfort and help her to feel free to express her feelings, whether positive or negative. I hoped that I could make her feel that I did not condemn her for being concerned about herself. Furthermore, I felt rather bold, almost guilty, for making the statement about concern for ourselves, for it was possible that I had misconstrued what she was trying to communicate.

The effectiveness of the intervention was obvious. I am firmly convinced that every medical-surgical nurse must be able to incorporate these principles into her approach to "nonpsychiatric" patients as well. In many situations she will encounter as intense emotional feelings as those in many psychiatric confrontations.

Mrs. M. began to ask other questions. She discussed the possibility of needing private duty nurses since her family would not be able to spend a great amount of time with her because of their distance from the hospital. I explained that she might be transferred to an intensive care unit where the nurses were especially trained. She said she was familiar with the small intensive care unit at the hospital where she worked. She expressed interest in seeing the unit at the medical center. Unfortunately, this could not be arranged because of time and the lack of communication between doctor and nurse.

At this point, she mentioned that she was a private patient but that, when she had arrived for admission, there were no semiprivate accommodations available and she had been placed on the ward. Initially, she said, she resented this. However, a few days later, she turned down the opportunity to transfer to a semiprivate room. She confided that the open ward provided her with a feeling of security — she could see the nurse all the time.

Mrs. M. then reverted to discussing the impending surgery (for removal of an acoustic neuroma). She expressed concern over her hair and said she had heard that her naturally curly hair would grow back straight. I reassured her that this was not so. She asked about the shaving which was to be done. I explained that this would be done in the operating room after she was under anesthesia. She said she was glad because she did not want any more people than necessary to see her without her hair.

Surgery was scheduled for the following day. Mrs. M. discussed the care of her valuables and belongings with me. She also mentioned that she had seen the priest and would see her family that evening; however, she said she did not want to see them before going for surgery in the morning. She was afraid that she might break down in front of them, something she did not want to do, although she said she did not object to crying in front of me.

DAY OF SURGERY

The morning of surgery, I visited Mrs. M. on the ward before she left for the operating room. I felt it would help her to discuss the possible outcomes of surgery, although I was severely handicapped by not knowing what the surgeon had told her. I approached the subject by asking if the doctor had come to talk with her. She replied that he had, and had told her that after surgery she would be completely deaf in the left ear and would have left-sided facial paralysis. She went on to say that she believed that the doctor had painted the picture as black as possible so she would not be too optimistic. However, Mrs. M. said, she realized rehabilitation would correct the defect within the span of a year. I did not pick up her cue because I did not feel it was an appropriate time to expand on that area.

In the preoperative care of this patient, I thought it was significant that she was concerned about being a "good" patient and about not boring me. Sometimes patients attempt to meet the needs of the nurse as they begin to realize they must depend on her for care at a later time. I hoped to impart to Mrs. M. a feeling that she could trust in me as her nurse, and that I would accept her behavior, whatever it might be. However, since she had worked with nurses in a hospital, she had heard many complain about patients who did not conform to their standards of behavior. I did feel she trusted me to some degree since she talked freely with me about some of her fears.

Her concern about her hair and facial appearance in the postoperative period and about people being unkind to deformed individuals reflected her concern about her body-image. It was quite obvious that this was a definite problem to her. I explained that just the back part of her head would be shaved. She felt somewhat relieved that she would not "look like Yul Brynner." I also mentioned that scarves and bandanas could be used to cover her head until her hair grew back. Mrs. M. talked about two people she knew who had had brain surgery. One was doing well; the other was still at home unable to walk without falling over to one side, suffered from facial "drooping," and had to have one of her eyelids sutured closed. However, Mrs. M went on, she was optimistic and had great faith in her doctor.

Psychologic preparation of Mrs. M was not entirely satisfactory. Better communication between doctors and nurses could have facilitated a more planned approach to help Mrs. M. accept her surgery. Her frequent episodes of crying, insomnia, and her loquaciousness were earmarks of a fairly high level of anxiety. Her efforts to reassure me that she took things as they came, that whatever would be would be, aroused my suspicions for she then usually broke into tears. Her attempts to reassure herself were short-lived.

Nursing care for Mrs. M. at this time needed to be directed toward reducing her anxiety. Considering the surgical procedure that Mrs. M. faced, the rapidity with which they informed her of her scheduled surgery, and the pessimistic picture painted by the physician, I believed that her reaction to these overwhelming circumstances was normal. At least, I think I would have reacted in much the same way.

Mrs. M. seemed to derive relief from anxiety from my efforts; for instance, she was able to go to sleep. I think she also derived a great deal of security from my presence while she waited in the operating room corridor; she said she was glad that I was with her. I expected her to make a satisfactory recovery since she exhibited interest in returning to work and her other activities. However, in more ways than one, man cannot predict the future.

POSTOPERATIVE CARE

Mrs. M. underwent a suboccipital craniectomy for the removal of an acoustic neuroma. For the first 12 hours postoperatively, Mrs. M.'s course was satisfactory. She did have a left facial palsy. However, while she was still in the recovery room, the surgeon noted that the decompression was firm. A ventricular tap showed increased cerebrospinal fluid pressure. Her blood pressure was rising. After removal of 40 cc. of cerebrospinal fluid from the ventricle, the decompression felt soft. But the therapeutic value of this procedure lasted only a few hours when, again, her blood pressure elevated. Destruction of the trigeminal nerve and the facial nerve was obvious at this point which meant that she had loss of sensation on the left side as well as facial paralysis, including lack of corneal reflex. It was obvious that her disability would be as the surgeon had predicted.

The immediate postoperative nursing care of Mrs. M. was primarily physical since she was semicomatose. Her pupils responded to light. She responded only to painful stimuli. I positioned her, did range of motion exercises with the permission of the doctor, gave mouth care and back care, kept a record of her intake and output, put ointment in her eye, gave needed medications, and checked the dressings for bleeding. I watched for signs and symptoms of increased intracranial hemorrhage, cerebral edema, hematoma, or meningitis. I noticed whether her pupils reacted to light and the state of their contraction or dilation, and I watched for changes in blood pressure, particularly increasing pressure. Since hyperthermia may result from a disturbance of the heat-controlling mechanism of the hypothalamus and brain stem, I took her temperature at regular intervals. And since respiratory collapse can occur with herniation of the cerebellar tonsils in association with an infratentorial tumor or with edema of the medulla oblongata, I observed her respirations very carefully.

About midmorning of Mrs. M.'s first postoperative day, she became extremely restless and attempted to sit up. Her blood pressure began to rise. The decompression was firm. The surgeon was notified and performed a lumbar puncture. At this point, Mrs. M. responded to pain.

Before the surgeon left the room, Mrs. M. showed signs of respiratory distress. Her breathing sounded as though there was an obstruction, but insertion of an airway did not relieve the distress. The surgeon performed a tracheostomy.

Mrs. M.'s care was important, but her family, too, needed care at this point — emotional support from the medical and nursing staffs. The family had been notified of the change in her condition and had arrived at the hospital early in the morning. I had the distinct advantage of knowing something about each member of the family through Mrs. M.'s desciptions of them before her surgery. Kay, her daughter-in-law, had recently graduated from a school of nursing. I planned to use her as the person to relate and interpret the patient's care and condition to other members of the family.

At first, members of the family seemed reticent about coming into Mrs. M.'s room. However, I reassured them that they were not getting in my way or interfering with her care in any way. I explained that many patients can hear what is said in the room even though they may not appear able to comprehend. Therefore, I suggested that it was wiser to not say anything that they did not want the patient to hear. I also suggested that they refrain from behavior that might distress the patient while they were in the room. The family responded amazingly well; they were quiet while they were with Mrs. M. Some members placed their hands on her forehead; others kissed her. However, all crying and discussion of the patient's condition was done outside of the room or in the lounge on the floor.

It must be frightening to see a patient with a Bird respirator attached to a tracheostomy, a tandem setup of intravenous fluid bottles, and tubes of different descriptions emerging from under the covers. Therefore, as each family member came to visit, I explained the various pieces of equipment. This had to be tempered to each individual. Mrs. M.'s sister appeared to be highly emotional, so I made the explanation to her very simple. Kay was interested in every aspect, and I tailored her explanation to her more highly technical level of understanding.

One of my responsibilities was to let the family realize they could talk to me about death. Some persons need a chance to be upset so that they can face the reality of what lies ahead. With support and guidance, a family may be able to talk more openly among themselves, and thereby gain strength from one another. Mr. M. had difficulty expressing anything. He appeared befuddled. As the day passed, and as I talked with him, he started to observe physical changes in Mrs. M. He said her arms were colder and he had not seen her move them. He mentioned she had no "temperature" in her body. He looked to me to negate his observations. I could only respond that the doctors were doing all they knew, but that it was in God's hands to decide. He shrugged his shoulders and left the room.

Mr. M. became more restless and upset as time passed. In view of his past medical history, I asked the physician to talk with the family and, perhaps, prescribe a sedative. He told the family that Mrs. M. had about a 20 percent chance of recovery.

Throughout the day, more and more family members arrived. One brought a relic she had purchased in St. Peter's Basilica in Rome. This was pinned to the patient's bed as requested. Each family member in his turn came to view Mrs. M. Some asked a few questions, others stood quietly and then left. A great amount of strength and consolation seemed to exist within the family circle.

By three o'clock in the afternoon, I noticed that none of the family had gone for lunch. I encouraged them to do so. Since they were reluctant, I suggested the hospital coffee shop, and I promised to call them if any changes occurred in Mrs. M.'s condition.

As the family members left to eat, Mrs. M.'s daughter came into the room and thanked me for caring for her mother. I was amazed and touched that, at a time of such emotional demand on her by her mother's illness and her father's grief, she would think of the nursing staff.

Mrs. M. died the next day. In retrospect, I think her family probably would have benefited if I could have spent more time with them even though they were a source of strength and comfort to one another. However, in the brief time I did have with them, I was able to help them to express some of their feelings. But, I do feel guilty about having to be so preoccupied with Mrs. M.'s physical care.

This experience was valuable to me. I had an opportunity to explore my feelings concerning death and the use of artificial means to maintain life. The doctor told me that he had prolonged Mrs. M.'s life by artificial means to give the family time to accept her approaching death. But, I cannot help but wonder if the members of her family awaken at night fearful, seeing, in distortion, all those strange tubes, noisy respirators, and other frightening-looking equipment. My feeling is that the medical team, inadvertently, makes death's reality obscure by making of it a public display of modern machinery.

The nurse frequently gives a reason for taking an action or making a statement. Note these reasons and think about alternate actions. List these and state your rationale.

Do you agree with the doctor's decision to artificially prolong Mrs. M.'s life?

What signs of changes in intracranial pressure were described?

Review the stages of grieving that the patient and family went through.

How would you evaluate her preoperative preparation?

Review selection #32 "Group Instruction in Preparation for Surgery," and list cues that might indicate a problem that you would want to pursue on a one-to-one basis.

47.

Pacemaker to the Rescue:
Its Use in the C.C.U.

Carole Shockey
Sandra Snow

If you are learning about pacemakers for the first time, you may wish to read selectively with the following questions in mind:

1. Why might a patient need a pacemaker after having a myocardial infarction?

2. How does a pacing catheter reach the heart where it does its work?

3. What complications might occur to the incision area? To the pacemaker and heart?

4. Why is a permanent pacemaker used and how is it inserted differently than a temporary one?

5. How do continuous, synchronized, and demand types of pacing differ?

If you are caring for a patient with a pacemaker in place, you can find detailed information on settings and monitoring changes.

Until the electronic cardiac pacemaker became widely available, the mortality rate for patients with third-degree atrioventricular block associated with myocardial infarction was extremely high. Today this device saves the lives of thousands of patients when the heart's own pacing system fails.

In 1958, electrical pacing was accomplished by means of a transvenous catheter into the heart. This is the method of choice today.

Third-degree heart block occurs in 2 to 10 per cent of patients with myocardial infarction. It may occur immediately after occlusion, but more frequently happens 24 to 72 hours later. It may last from a few hours to many weeks, or it may be permanent, depending on the site and extent of the infarction and the degree of collateral circulation that develops.[1] Usually, various drugs are given to try to prevent it. Some authorities advocate inserting a pacing catheter only after the drugs have been tried without success.

The pacing catheter is bipolar or unipolar, silastic-covered, and approximately 125 cm. in length. Insertion is sometimes done in the coronary-care unit, but more often in the X-ray department or the cardiac catheterization lab. Fluoroscopy and cardiac monitoring are used to help guide the catheter to its destination. It is inserted — under local anesthesia — either through the external jugular vein or the brachiocephalic vein, and is passed through the right atrium and the tricuspid valve. The electrode at its tip is lodged against the endocardium at the apex of the right ventricle between the trabeculae carneae cordis. To test the security of placement, the patient is moved to different positions and performs respiratory exercises.

The catheter is connected to a small demand or set-rate pacemaker with its own battery power source that is attached to the patient's arm or chest.[2] If electrode placement seems satisfactory, lateral and A-P chest X-rays are taken to check the catheter's position and provide a comparison in follow-up studies of position. ECG leads are connected to the bedside monitor, and a grounding wire may be taped to the patient's skin. (Defibrillating equipment is kept on hand in case of ventricular fibrillation.)

Two settings are made on the pacemaker. First, the milliamperage threshold potential of the patient is found by determining the minimal amount of milliamperes (ma.) that will produce cardiac response. For most patients, the threshold potential is 0.5 to 0.75 ma.[3] The pacemaker is set at two ma. higher — for example, at 2.5 ma. for the 0.5 patient.

Second, the pacing rate (heart rate) control is set, usually at 70 to 75 impulses per minute. If transient ectopic tachycardia occurs, the rate may be increased to help convert the heartbeat to normal. The increased rate is maintained only for short intervals, however, for it's thought that prolonged artificially stimulated tachycardia may add an extra burden to the already ischemic myocardium and produce cardiogenic shock.

---

[1] For a capsule review of heart block, see page 306.

[2] This miniaturized model has replaced the bedside pacemaker in most hospitals because of its safety and convenience. Accidental electric shock cannot occur, and the pacemaker is shielded from electrical equipment that might interfere with its pacing impulses. All electrical equipment in the area is carefully and adequately grounded.

[3] Some authorities recommend a threshold above 1 ma. or 1.5 ma.

WHAT HAPPENS IN HEART BLOCK

The atria, atrioventricular (AV) node, and the ventricles all have the potential to act as the heart's pacemaker. Normally, however, the sino-atrial (SA) node dominates because it discharges impulses at a faster rate than any of the other sites. If for some reason the rate of one or more of the other sites increases beyond that of the SA node, these impulses interfere with or block the SA node impulses.

In AV block following myocardial infarction, the blood supply to the AV node is so obstructed that ischemia or edema prevents functioning of the nodal fibers. Impulses arising from the SA node are blocked by these diseased fibers, and "heart block" is said to occur.

Occlusion of the right coronary artery is almost always the cause of heart block following myocardial infarction; for in 90 per cent of patients, a branch of this vessel supplies the AV node and the bundle of His. A large transeptal infarction usually causes extensive disruption; a diaphragmatic infarction causes transient disruption.

When the right coronary artery (or a branch to the AV node) is involved, the heart block usually lasts from 7 to 14 days, provided adequate tissue perfusion is afforded by the collateral circulation. Acute extensive infarction of the interventricular septum usually produces permanent heart block. Ischemia with reactionary edema of the AV node may produce heart block of only two to three days' duration. Persistent hypotension and shock caused by AV block are almost always fatal.

The patient on a pacemaker is usually monitored for a minimum of three days, preferably in the coronary-care unit. Vital signs, urinary output, and level of alertness are checked frequently to be sure adequate cardiac output is maintained. If any marked changes occur, the physician is notified immediately. If supportive oxygen therapy is needed, it is administered by mask or nasal cannula. The catheter incision is treated like any other surgical wound. (Sterile technique is used with dressing changes, and the area is observed for signs of phlebitis.) Intermittent hyperventilation, turning, and passive cardiac exercises are done routinely, and antibiotics are often given prophylactically. Anticoagulant therapy is not usually undertaken.

Complications that may occur include malposition of the catheter electrode, cardiac perforation by the electrode, equipment failure, bacteremia, phlebitis, and ventricular fibrillation. Malfunction of the pacemaker poses a special danger for this reason: Its impulses cause a pacing artifact, or blip, to appear on the monitor and the ECG as an upward deflection directly ahead of the QRS complex. The monitor's alarm system reacts to this artifact as it does to the complex. As long as the artifact continues to appear, the monitor will not sound an alarm. Thus if a pacemaker continues to send its impulses after a patient's heart has ceased responding, the patient may succumb without triggering the warning buzzer. The nurse, therefore, observes the screen to see if the ventricular complex follows, or if pacing occurs haphazardly. She also checks the patient's pulse to determine if the beat is conducted to the radial artery.

If a patient's heart has not returned to sinus rhythm after 7 to 10 days, a permanent pacemaker may be provided. The temporary catheter is removed, and a permanent catheter is passed through the external jugular vein to the right ventricle and positioned in the same manner as was the temporary catheter. It is then connected to a battery-powered pacemaker about the size of a pack of cigarettes. This unit is implanted subcutaneously in pectoralis muscle near the patient's right axilla. (Occasionally the batteries are implanted separately in corresponding tissue of the patient's left side to accommodate a particular patient's needs.)

The patient is taught to check his pulse daily and to notify his doctor immediately if any vertigo, syncope, pulse rate variation, visual change, or chest pain occurs. An increase in pulse rate may indicate that the batteries are weakening. Their condition may then be checked by radioscopic examination. (A functioning battery appears as an opaque unit, a failing battery as a radiolucent coil.) Though pacemaker batteries are designed to last five years, most doctors advocate replacing them every two or three years as a safety measure.

There are three kinds of permanent pacemakers: continuous (fixed rate), synchronized (variable rate), and demand (stand-by). The continuous pacemaker functions at a predetermined rate and completely controls the pacing of the heart. The synchronized type acts as a bridge between the sino-atrial (SA) node and the right ventricle when the atrioventricular (AV) node is not functioning. It is usually set so that if the sinus rate increases to 110, the pacer blocks alternate beats. If the SA node becomes diseased, this pacemaker takes over and paces the heart permanently. The demand type functions only when the heart rate drops below a prefixed level or when the depolarization interval of the heartbeat is too prolonged.

Both the continuous and synchronized pacemakers have a threatening complication: Competition may develop between their impulses and the heart's owm rhythm that may conflict with the pacing artifact and ultimately cause ventricular fibrillation. The demand pacemaker has the disadvantage that because it may seldom be in use, there is always the question as to whether it is operational. However, a physician can check its status periodically by several external methods.

For all models, infrequent complications include electrode breakage, wire breakage, and the formation of scar tissue at the site of the implanted electrode. (Scar tissue is nonconductive.) Recently, the use of a new metal alloy called

Elgiloy has decreased the incidence of electrode breakage; and relocation of battery implants from abdominal to subpectoral pockets has decreased wire breakage by 12 per cent.

Research has not yet produced a way to provide a reliable power source other than to replace the batteries by periodic surgery. The use of externally rechargeable batteries, body fuel cells, and atomic-powered batteries is being explored. A new system of emergency pacing at the bedside, called magnetic guidance, is also in the experimental stage.

To summarize: Demand cardiac pacing is presently the treatment of choice in complete, transient, or permanent AV block. But there is much that science still has to explore in this area. Constant study and continued close cooperation among patient, nurse, physician, and manufacturer will be necessary to solve this complex challenge in bioelectronics.

Now that you have completed this article, write and discuss specific answers to the questions on page 304.

48.

What Stress Can Do To You

Walter McQuade

Think about how you react to stress. This article will give you historical and current ideas on stress and its reactions. Underline points that interest you and discuss them with your peers.

It has long been a matter of common intuition that bottled-up anger can crack the bottle, prolonged strain can make people sick. This old folklore now has considerable scientific support. Stress might be defined as the body's involuntary reactions to the demanding life that we Americans choose—or that chooses us.

These reactions are rooted deep in the prehistory of the human species. Early man survived in a brutal world because, along with an elaborate brain, he had the mechanisms of instantaneous, unthinking physical response when in danger. Picture a primitive man, many thousands of years ago, lying in the sun in front of his cave after the hunt, digesting. Suddenly he felt the cool shadow of a predatory carnivore, stalking. Without thinking, he reacted with a mighty surge of bodily resources. Into his blood flashed adrenal secretions that mustered strength in the form of both sugar and stored fats to his muscles and brain, instantly mobilizing full energy, and stimulating pulse, respiration, and blood pressure. His digestive processes turned off at once so that no energy was diverted from meeting the threat. His coagulation chemistry immediately prepared to resist wounds with quick clotting. Red cells poured from the spleen into the stepped-up blood circulation to help the respiratory system take in oxygen and cast off carbon dioxide as this ancestral man clubbed at the prowling beast, or scuttled safely back into his cave.

A COOL MEMO FROM A V.P.

Today, say stress researchers, a man in a business suit still reacts, within his skin, in much the same chemical way. He does so although today's threat is more likely to be in the abstract, for example, a cool memo from a vice president of the corporation: "The chairman wants a study of the savings possible in merging your division with warehousing and relocating to South Carolina."

Flash go the hormones into the blood; up goes the pulse beat—but the manager who receives the memo can neither fight physically nor flee. Instead his first tendency is to stall, which only induces guilt, before he plunges into a battle fought with no tangible weapons heavier than paper clips. Under his forced calm builds repressed rage without any adequate target—except himself.

If he is the kind of hard-driving, competitive perfectionist whom many corporations prize, and if this kind of stress pattern is chronic, the stress experts will tell you that he is a prime candidate for an early coronary (an even likelier candidate than American men in general, whose chances of having a heart attack before age sixty are one in five). If not a coronary, it may be migraine, ulcers, asthma, ulcerative colitis, or even the kind of scalp itch James V. Forrestal developed as he began to give way to interior pressure. Or perhaps a collision on the road—stressed people are more accident-prone.

Chronic strain is so common that there are conventional ways of fighting back. Millions of pills repose in desk drawers, ready to foster calmness or energy. The trouble with them, say the doctors, is that after the calm or the uplift there usually comes a period of depression. Martinis may be better, although they too involve dangers. Some people under stress try to vent their repressed anger in polite violence at a driving range or bowling alley, or by chopping wood or throwing themselves at ocean waves breaking on the beach. But the violent exercisers had better be careful of contracting another common stress symptom, low back pain.

Marriages have to accept a lot of stress, both in hurtful words and yet another symptom, temporary impotence. If a man coming under job stress has been on an anticholesterol diet he had better stay on it, but the competitive strain on him will be upping his serum cholesterol, whatever he eats. In broad terms, man the victorious predator now preys internally on himself.

LOST CONSOLATIONS

Why has stress become such a problem in today's world of mass-manufactured comforts and conveniences? For most people in industrial nations, after all, life is in many respects a lot easier than it was for their ancestors. Perhaps the answer, or at least part of the answer, is that modern societies have to a great extent lost the supports that helped people in earlier times endure toil, hardship, and suffering—religious faith, sustaining frameworks of tradition and custom, a sense of place in the social order, a sense of worth derived from the exercise of craftsmanship, and awareness that toil, hardship, and suffering were likewise endured by the other members of the same community and the same social class. In the twentieth century the great increase in physical abundance has been accompanied by swift and deep erosion of these intangible sources of consolation and support.

Particularly destructive of the individual's sense of security have been the side effects of one of the industrial world's most precious products—social mobility. This bright trophy of our times has its deeply etched dark side. Social mobility has weakened the sense of belonging to a class, the sense of having a place in the social order. More important, social mobility implies that success depends on merit alone, and to the extent that a society believes in such correlation, individual bread-winners are thrust into an endless competition in which losing or lagging can be interpreted as a sign of personal inadequacy.

Stress, then, is rampant not in rural or in underdeveloped countries, but in the great urban centers of the industrialized world. And it is not surprising that external threats to the community tend to decrease individual stress rather than increasing it. In England, for example, two prime indexes of stress, alcoholism and suicide, declined markedly during World War II.

As a recognized factor in disease, stress is very much a product of the twentieth century. When it was still but vaguely recognized forty years ago, the medical historian Henry E. Sigerist foresaw its importance. Every epoch, he observed, has its characteristic ailments. "It seems as though the powers that ordain the style for and stamp their impress upon a certain epoch affect even disease." He pointed out that the Middle Ages were dominated by ills of the common people such as the great plague, leprosy, and the epidemic neuroses, which appeared in the sixth to the fourteenth centuries. The disease that characterized the Renaissance was syphilis, an infection incurred not passively but as a result of an individual act. "In the discordant Baroque era, the foreground is occupied by diseases which might be called deficiency diseases like camp-fever, scurvy and ergotism on the one hand and on the other by diseases which might be called luxury diseases like gout, dropsy and hypochondriasis." Tuberculosis and similar ailments characterized the romantic period, "while the 19th century, with its tremendously increased industrialization, the development of great cities and the accelerated life tempo, brought about industrial diseases, general nervousness and neuroses of many kinds."

THE SEEDS AND THE TERRAIN

Medicine, too, has its epochs. Until late in the nineteenth century, the leading doctors were generalists, devoutly concerned with the "whole man." According to Sir William Osler, the famous Canadian clinician, "It is much more important to know what sort of a patient has a disease than what sort of a disease a patient has." Claude Bernard, the most renowned of nineteenth-century French physicians, maintained that diseases were resisted by a person's central equilibrium, his *milieu interieur*; the germs were all about, like seeds blown by the wind., but did not take root in his "terrain" unless he had already been weakened.

After the middle of the nineteenth century, however, the medical world's focus of attention began to shift from the patient to the disease. Pasteur and other great scientists achieved glorious successes in identifying harmful micro-organisms, and medicine knocked off one disease after another. Many doctors came to consider the question of the patient's receptivity to illness almost quaint, except in such obvious conditions of weakness as severe malnutrition. By 1943, Dr. Flanders Dunbar of Columbia University-Presbyterian Hospital in New York was able to point out that of the most common dangerous illnesses in America fifty years earlier—infections such as scarlet fever and typhoid—not one was still on the list of the ten most common causes of mortality and morbidity.

Yet the hospitals were still full. It almost seemed that man was inventing new chronic diseases to replace the old infections. The realization sent some medical practitioners and researchers back to the whole-man concept. In the vanguard was Dr. Harold G. Wolff of New York Hospital-Cornell Medical Center, who wrote that in infectious disease "the presence of the micro-organism, however indispensable, is not sufficient as the cause of illness. . .In a sense, disease is a reaction to rather than an effect of noxious forces."

Through painstaking observation and accumulation of case histories, Dunbar, Wolff, and other investigators were able to demonstrate that many persons who had become vulnerable to certain organisms shared not only physical but also psychological characteristics. This was especially true in chronic conditions such as eczema, gastric ulcer, diabetes, arthritis, migraine, asthma, and ulcerative colitis. The researchers decided that the Victorian novelists had been excellent intuitive diagnosticians in discerning that people who had been through periods of severe emotional upset, such as a broken love affair, or depression caused by the death of a beloved mate, were especially vulnerable to pulmonary tuberculosis. More recently a high incidence of cancer has been found in the same circumstances, but the evidence is less convincing, so far, than with TB. Some studies indicate also that vulnerabilities shift as social patterns change. For example, peptic ulcers used to be primarily a woman's ailment. One retrospective medical study reveals that from 1850 to 1900 close to seven out of every ten patients with perforated peptic ulcers were women. But from 1920 to 1940 nine out of every ten were men. Since mid-century the incidence of ulcers in women has been on the rise again.

A growing accumulation of evidence indicates that a great many bodily ills that afflict human beings are partly psychosomatic in nature. For example, a period of mental depression affects a patient's nasal mucous membranes, making him somewhat more vulnerable to virus infections. As one doctor observed, "You don't have to be depressed to get a cold, but it helps."

Some very different chronic illnesses have been interlinked. The *Journal of Chronic Diseases* several years ago published a paper entitled "Why Do Wives with Rheumatoid Arthritis Have Husbands with Peptic Ulcer?" The answer was a summary of research revealing the existence of a particular type of hostility in such marriages. The wife, conditioned by early childhood, had a yearning for high public esteem, an ambition that her husband could not, or would not, enable her to gratify. Frequently, the husband was of the common ulcer type, in strong need of emotional support, which the wife, because of her resentment, did not provide.

Aggression is likely to be clearer in close business relationships than in marriages, but still not simple. Dr. Sidney Cobb, one of the authors of the paper on arthritic wives and ulcerous husbands, recently noted in conversation that many a quietly aggressive executive unconsciously picks an ulcer-prone assistant, sensing that the assistant can be prodded into anxious action just by the boss's failure to say good morning.

DISCOVERING THE UBIQUITOUS

A pioneer investigator into the implications of stress was Dr. Hans Selye, a Canadian who has become the world's acknowledged authority on his subject. Selye, now sixty-four, defines stress as the nonspecific response of the body to any demand made on it. He maintains that stress went unstudied in detail for centuries simply because it had always been so common.

Selye explains that when the brain signals the attack of a stressor—which could be either a predatory beast or a threatening memorandum—the adrenal and pituitary glands produce the hormones ACTH, cortisone, and cortisol, which stimulate protective bodily reactions. If the stress is a fresh wound, the blood rushes irritants to seal it off; if the stress is a broken bone, swelling occurs around the break. The pro-inflammatory hormones are balanced by anti-inflammatory hormones, which prevent the body from reacting so strongly that the reaction causes more harm than the invasion.

ENERGY THAT CAN'T BE REPLENISHED

So the initial reaction to any kind of stress is alarm. It is followed by an instantaneous rallying of the body's defenses. The fight is on—even if the body, in effect, is just fighting the mind. If the threat recedes or is overcome, stability returns. But if the attack is prolonged, deterioration sets in, as the defense system gradually wears down. Selye calls this process the General Adaptation Syndrome, and it is recognized in the field as a brilliant concept.

Stress is not only a killer, Selye teaches, but also a drastic aging force. Different men have different hereditary capacities to withstand stress, but once each man's "adaptation energy" has been expended, there is no way yet known to replenish it.

Selye likens each man's supply of life energy to deep deposits of oil; once the man has summoned it up and burned it in the form of adaptation energy, it is gone—and so, soon, is he. If he picks a high-stress career, he spends his portion fast and ages fast. "There are two ages," says Selye, "one which is chronological, an absolute, and the other which is biologic and is your effective age. It is astonishing how the two can differ."

A QUEERLY CONTEMPORARY QUALITY

Stress research in the U.S. centers on heart disease, and for good reason. Cardiovascular ailments such as coronary heart disease now take an appalling annual toll in lives of American men in vigorous middle age. Of the 700,000 people who died from coronary heart disease in the U.S. last year, almost 200,000 were under sixty-five.

Yet until this century heart disease was virtually unknown anywhere in the world, and as late as the 1920's it was still fairly rare in the U.S. Dr. Paul Dudley White, the eminent cardiologist, recalls that in the first two years after he set up his practice in 1912 he saw only three or four coronary patients. The queerly contemporary quality of heart disease cannot be attributed to the ignorance of earlier doctors. As far back as the time of Hippocrates, most afflictions were described well enough to be recognizable today from surviving records. A convincing description of heart disease, however, was not entered in medical records until late in the eighteenth century. John R. P. French, Jr., an austere and plainspoken psychologist at the institute, says that the known risk factors do not come close to accounting for the incidence of the disease. He maintains that "if you could perfectly control cholesterol, blood pressure, smoking, glucose level, serum uric acid, and so on, you would have controlled only about one-fourth of the coronary heart disease." There is little solid evidence, he adds, "to show that programs of exercise substantially reduce the incidence of coronary heart disease or substantially reduce some of the risk factors."

To a great extent, argues French, the problem is the job. "The stresses of today's organizations can pose serious threats to the phsyical and psychological well-being of organization members. When a man dies or becomes disabled by a heart attack, the organization may be as much to blame as is the man and his family."

Other occupational stresses found by the survey included insecurity asso-ciated with having to venture outside normal job boundaries; difficult bosses or subordinates; worry over carrying responsibility for other people; the lack of a feeling of participation in decisions governing their jobs—a malaise, adds Dr. French, that distinctly lowers productivity.

THE CORONARY TYPE

It is not a new observation that some people are more subject to stress than others. Sir William Osler lived too early to see many coronary cases, but he left a shrewd description of the angina type. "It is not the delicate, neurotic person who is prone to angina," he commented, "but the robust, the vigorous in mind and body, the keen and ambitious man, the indicator of whose engine is always at 'full speed ahead'. . .the well set man of from forty-five to fifty-five years of age, with military bearing, iron gray hair, and florid complexion."

This Osler quotation is a favorite of two California cardiologists, Meyer Friedman and Ray H. Rosenman, who are among the country's leading students of stress. In the past seventeen years they and their staff at the Harold Brunn Institute of Mount Zion Hospital in San Francisco have spent thousands of hours and hundreds of thousands of research dollars building up an impressive case that behavior patterns and stress are principal culprits in the high incidence of coronary heart attacks among middle-aged Americans—and that personality differences are of vital importance.

In studying reactions to stress, Friedman and Rosenman gradually came to the conviction that people can be divided into two major types, which they designate A and B. Type A, the coronary-prone type, is characterized by intense drive, aggressiveness, ambition, competitiveness, pressure for getting things done, and the habit of pitting himself against the clock. He also exhibits visible restlessness. Type B may be equally serious, but is more easygoing in manner, seldom becomes impatient, and takes more time to enjoy leisure. He does not feel driven by the clock. He is not preoccupied with social achievement, is less competitive, and even speaks in a more modulated style. Most people are mixtures of Type A and Type B characteristics, but a trained interviewer can spot one pattern or the other as predominant.

A RATHER GRIM CHUCKLE

The extreme Type A is a tremendously hard worker, a perfectionist, filled with brisk self-confidence, decisiveness, resolution. He never evades. He is the man who, while waiting in the office of his cardiologist or dentist, is on the telephone making business calls. His wife is certain he drives himself too hard, and she may be a little in awe of him. The world is a deadly serious game, and he is out to amass points enough to win.

He speaks in staccato, and has a tendency to end his sentences in a rush. He frequently sighs faintly between words, but never in anxiety, because that state is strange to him. He is seldom out sick. He rarely goes to doctors, almost never to psychiatrists. He is unlikely to get an ulcer. He is rarely interested in money except as a token of the game, but the higher he climbs, the more he considers himself underpaid.

On the debit side, he is often a little hard to get along with. His chuckle is rather grim. He does not drive people who work under him as hard as he drives himself, but he has little time to waste with them. He wants their respect, not their affection. Yet in some ways he is more sensitive than the milder Type B. He hates to fire anyone and will go to great lengths to avoid it. Sometimes the only way he can resolve such a situation is by mounting a crisis. If he himself has ever been fired, it was probably after a personality clash.

Type A, surprisingly, probably goes to bed earlier most nights than Type B, who will get interested in something irrelevant to his career and sit up late, or simply socialize. Type A is precisely on time for appointments and expects the same from other people. He smokes cigarettes, never a pipe. Headwaiters learn not to keep him waiting for a table reservation; if they do, they lose him. They like him because he doesn't linger over his meals, and doesn't complain about quality. He will usually salt the meal before he tastes it. He's never sent a bottle of wine back in his life. Driving a car, Type A is not reckless, but does reveal anger when a slower driver ahead delays him.

Type A's are not much for exercise; they claim they have too little time for it. When they do play golf, it is fast through. They never return late from vacation. Their desk tops are clean when they leave the office at the end of each day.

AN UNRECOGNIZED SICKNESS

Type B's differ little in background or ability from A's, and may be quietly urgent, but they are more reasonable men. Unlike Type A, Type B is hard to needle into anger. Friedman says, "A's have no respect for B's, but the smart B uses an A. The great salesmen are A's. The corporation presidents are usually B's."

What is most tragic of all in this picture of hopeful, driving, distorting energy is that the Type A's are from two to three times more likely than the Type B's to get coronary heart disease in middle age. In all of Sinclair Lewis' pitiless characterizations of the go-getting American businessman of another era, there is nothing so devastating as these doctors' cool, clincial statistics. Rosenman about the Type A condition: "It is a sickness, although it is not yet recognized as such."

The test program that Friedman and Rosenman offer as their strongest body of evidence was undertaken in 1960 with substantial backing from the National Institutes of Health. A total of 3,500 male subjects aged thirty-nine to fifty-nine, with no known history of heart disease, were interviewed and classified as Type

A or Type B. So far, 257 of the test group—who are roughly half A's and half B's—have developed coronary heart disease. Seventy percent of the victims have been Type A's.

Dr. Roseman reported any B whose level of cholesterol and other fatty acids was within normal limits "had complete immunity to coronary heart disease, irrespective of his high-fat, cholesterol diet, family history, or his habits of smoking or his lack of exercising."

What creates a Type B or Type A? These cardiologists do not profess to know the complete answer yet. But to them it is obvious that both heredity and environment are involved. A's are naturally attracted toward careers of aggressiveness and deadline pressure. American life today, Friedman and Rosenman observe, offers plenty of these. What Type A's need but cannot easily achieve is restraint, says Dr. Friedman, who himself suffered a heart attack in 1967.

LAST WORDS OF A GREAT MAN

Now that even cardiologists are beginning to believe heart disease can be traced to unrelenting competiveness and baffled fury, will a wave of concern over stress sweep over this hypochondriacal country, to match the widespread interest in jogging and polyunsaturated oils? Quite likely. There is nothing more fascinating to the layman than folklore finally validated by reputable scientists. A murmur of assent rises faintly from the past. When the great Pasteur lay in terminal illness, in 1895, he reflected once again on his long scientific disagreement with Claude Bernard. Pasteur's dying words were: "Bernard was right. The microbe is nothing, the terrain is everything."

Describe a stress reaction of your own that you experienced recently. Compare this to the description of the cave man's reaction.

List the signs for "A" and "B." Are you an "A" or "B" reactor? Is nursing a stressful occupation?

List some of the possible causes of the problem of stress today. How has social mobility affected security and stress?

What was the effect of World War II on alcoholism and suicide in England? Why? What similar examples of external threats in this country today can you give that may decrease stress to the individual?

List the ages and characteristic ailments given in the article.

How do your chronologic and biologic ages differ? What is the significance to you?

INDEX

The index cross references to patient problems, situations or subjects within selections. Numbers refer to selections instead of pages. This should be used along with the table of contents.

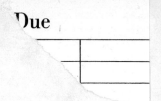

Due